CALVERT'S DESCRIPTIVE PHONETICS

Third Edition

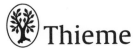
Thieme

CALVERT'S DESCRIPTIVE PHONETICS

Third Edition

Pamela G. Garn-Nunn, Ph.D.
Professor
Undergraduate Coordinator
School of Speech-Language Pathology and Audiology
The University of Akron
Akron, OH

James M. Lynn, Ph.D.
Professor of Audiology
Associate Dean
College of Fine and Applied Arts
The University of Akron
Akron, OH

Thieme

New York • Stuttgart

Thieme Medical Publishers, Inc.
333 Seventh Ave.
New York, NY 10001

Director, Production and Manufacturing: Anne Vinnicombe
Production Editor: Becky Dille
Marketing Director: Phyllis Gold
Sales Manager: Ross Lumpkin
Chief Financial Officer: Peter van Woerden
President: Brian D. Scanlan
Compositor: Compset, Inc.
Printer: Maple-Vail Book Manufacturing Group
Library of Congress Cataloging-in-Publication Data

Important note: Medical knowledge is ever-changing. As new research and clinical experience broaden our knowledge, changes in treatment and drug therapy may be required. The authors and editors of the material herein have consulted sources believed to be reliable in their efforts to provide information that is complete and in accord with the standards accepted at the time of publication. However, in the view of the possibility of human error by the authors, editors, or publisher, of the work herein, or changes in medical knowledge, neither the authors, editors, or publisher, nor any other party who has been involved in the preparation of this work, warrants that the information contained herein is in every respect accurate or complete, and they are not responsible for any errors or omissions or for the results obtained from use of such information. Readers are encouraged to confirm the information contained herein with other sources. For example, readers are advised to check the product information sheet included in the package of each drug they plan to administer to be certain that the information contained in this publication is accurate and that changes have not been made in the recommended dose or in the contraindications for administration. This recommendation is of particular importance in connection with new or infrequently used drugs.

Some of the product names, patents, and registered designs referred to in this book are in fact registered trademarks or proprietary names even though specific reference to this fact is not always made in the text. Therefore, the appearance of a name without designation as proprietary is not to be construed as a representation by the publisher that it is in the public domain.

Printed in the United States of America
5 4 3 2 1
TMP ISBN 1-58890-019-3
GTV ISBN 3 13 608004 1

CONTENTS

PREFACE

This third edition of *Calvert's Descriptive Phonetics* contains both similarities to and differences from previous editions. The most obvious difference, of course, is that Donald Calvert, the original author, is no longer with us. Jim Lynn and I assumed the authorship with full recognition of the quality of previous editions and a determination to maintain it. We have attempted to follow Dr. Calvert's lead in writing a text that would be most useful to a wide variety of readers, but especially to those who are studying to help others work on their speech: speech-language pathologists, teachers of children who are hearing impaired or deaf, teachers of English as a second language (ESL), and coaches of dramatics and diction. We hope that students and instructors in these specialties will find the text informative, comprehensive, and useful.

Although the content areas covered remain the same as in previous editions, we have made some organizational changes and added new information. In particular, Chapter 1 and the chapters on dialectic variations and acoustic phonetics have been extensively rewritten. Information about distinctive features has also been added. Additionally, we changed the order of presentation for vowels and consonants so that the chapter on vowels now precedes the chapter on consonants. This was a choice based on teaching experience with a large number of undergraduate students over the years. Otherwise, the emphases of this text remain much the same.

This book is designed primarily as a text for students beginning the study of phonetics. Exercises are included at the end of each chapter to help the student understand and learn the information. Further practice in phonetic transcription may be gained through use of the workbook that is a companion to this text: *Calvert's Descriptive Phonetics Transcription Workbook*, third edition.

The pronunciations in this book are those most commonly associated with what has previously been referred to as standard American English (SAE) or general American English (GAE). In this text, we will discuss mainstream American English and its dialectic variations. In Chapter 9, mainstream AE will serve as the reference for discussing a number of dialectic variations. We wish to stress that no one dialectic variation of English has an inherent value in and of itself. Based on the most recent studies by linguists, a variety of dialects can be found within our borders. This book has been designed as an introductory text in phonetics and we felt that students should be made aware of key regional and cultural dialects.

To all those at Thieme and at the University of Akron who were involved in bringing this edition into being, we extend our thanks. In particular, we're grateful to the students in our undergraduate phonetics classes of 2000 and 2001. They "test drove" earlier versions of the manuscript for us and gave us needed input. And, to our graduate assistant proofreaders, Kristine Corcoran and Jamie Harding, thanks for all the time and eyestrain!

P.G.G-N.
J.M.L.

FOREWORD TO THE INSTRUCTOR

This edition has been designed for college-level students as an introductory text. No previous knowledge of phonetics, and only a rudimentary knowledge of anatomy, physiology, and physics, is prerequisite. Each chapter begins with an outline, followed by text. New terms are highlighted when they are introduced. Each chapter concludes with review vocabulary and exercises designed to help the student learn and understand chapter content. Although we have attempted to help the student learn as much from reading the text as possible, there is no substitute for a course that includes lecture, examples, and multiple opportunities for transcription practice. Instructors may find that they wish to use all or only parts of this book, depending on course focus and content.

Our primary purpose is to give students the opportunity to

1. Develop listening and analytic skills
2. Gain knowledge and understanding of speech
3. Be introduced to some of the specialty areas of phonetics
4. Have access to resource materials that may be helpful in applying this knowledge

The following list shows these objectives matched with chapter designations.

1. Develop Listening and Analytic Skills
   - Phonetic transcription, broad and narrow International Phonetic Alphabet (IPA): Chapters 1–6
   - Indication speech rhythm features: Chapter 6
   - Analysis of how speech units are produced: Chapters 2–6
2. Gain Knowledge and Understanding of Speech
   - Nature of orthographic systems: Chapter 1
   - Anatomy and physiologic processes of speech production: Chapter 2
   - Categorization of vowels and consonants according to traditional and distinctive feature classifications: Chapter 3
   - Categorization of vowels by place and height of tongue elevation: Chapters 3–4
   - Categorization of consonants by place, manner, and voicing: Chapters 3, 5
   - Influences of phonetic context and coarticulation: Chapter 6
   - Relation of speech rhythm and pronunciation: Chapter 6
   - Acoustic phonetics: Chapter 7
   - Dialectic variations: Chapter 8
   - Relation of acoustic parameters to oral positions: Chapters 3–7
   - Vocabulary associated with phonetics: Chapters 1–9

3. Be Introduced to Specialty Areas of Phonetics
   - Physiologic phonetics: Chapters 2–5
   - American English pronunciations: Chapters 1–6, 8
   - Multicultural considerations and dialectic variations: Chapters 4, 5, 8
   - Acoustic phonetics: Chapter 7
   - Applications of phonetics: Chapter 9
4. Have Access to Resource Material for Reference
   - Formation of primary American English phonemes: Chapters 3–5
   - Spellings for primary phonemes: Chapters 1, 3–5
   - Word examples of phonemes in all positions: Chapters 3–5
   - Examples of phonemes in sentences: Chapters 4, 5
   - Word sets contrasting similar or often confused phonemes: Chapters 4–5
   - General American symbol system for reading and spelling: Chapter 1

You will notice that most objectives are not confined to just one chapter. Even in Chapter 1 we introduce students to IPA consonant and vowel symbols, returning to them repeatedly, especially in Chapters 3, 4, and 5. Basic knowledge underlying physiologic phonetics is found in Chapter 2 and reiterated in later chapters as consonant and vowel symbols are introduced. After basic transcription skills are developed, students can learn about advanced narrow transcription in Chapter 6 and acoustic phonetics in Chapter 7. Further application of basic knowledge can be developed through reading and studying Chapters 8 and 9, which cover dialectic variations and applied phonetics, respectively.

For those instructors who want to emphasize transcription practice, there is also a workbook, *Calvert's Descriptive Phonetics Transcription Workbook,* third edition, which accompanies this text. We revised the workbook to help students develop their transcription skills, beginning in each chapter with recognition exercises, followed by discrimination exercises and finally, actual transcription. An instructional CD covering introductory, vowel, and consonant workbook exercises, is also available for the workbook. Whether you use this textbook by itself or in conjunction with the workbook, we hope that you find it a helpful teaching and learning tool.

CHAPTER 1

INTRODUCTION

ALPHABETIC LETTERS, SPEECH SOUNDS, AND THE INTERNATIONAL
PHONETIC ALPHABET
BASIC TERMS AND DEFINITIONS
REVIEW VOCABULARY
EXERCISES

Imagine that you are a game show contestant with a chance to win a huge cash
prize. You have a partner in this contest with whom you must agree in order to win
the money. What do you have to agree on? Just the pronunciation and meaning
of words in a foreign language that neither you nor your partner knows anything
about. According to the game show rules, you and your partner (separately) will
view a 1-hour videotape of people teaching vocabulary and phrases in this language.
Each of you must determine the meaning and pronunciation of as many words as
possible. After the hour of videotape viewing, you and your partner will have 15
minutes to compare notes. The more words you can identify, the more money you
will win. Sounds reasonably easy, right? Armed with note-taking supplies, you each
watch the tape and record word pronunciations and meanings. You then sit down
together to compare notes. You discover a problem. You see, your partner is from
Russia, and her notes look totally different from yours. For the word in the unfamiliar language that seems to mean "hello," you wrote *hi,* and your partner wrote
Хай. Now what? (Remember, you have only 15 minutes to agree on as many words
as possible.)

Does that example seem too far-fetched to you? Well, try this next one. Imagine
that you teach voice and diction to students majoring in oral communications.
Another teacher tells you that his ESL students (who speak English as a second,
rather than first, or native, language) are having trouble pronouncing the English *a.*
"Which *a?*" you ask. The one in *apple?* In *bake?* Or maybe the one in *calm?*

Obviously, when we depend on different orthographic systems, communication
can be a problem. Each of us learned **orthography** (the accurate or accepted
spelling of words using alphabet symbols) early in our schooling. But different languages can use different alphabets. Some sounds occur in one language but not in
another (e.g., German does not have *th* sounds, but English lacks the pharyngeal
sounds of other languages).

"Well," you reply, "then let's use diacritical markings like a dictionary does." That might very well solve our confusion over "Which *a?*" provided (1) we speak English and (2) we understand those diacritical markings (e.g., long *a,* or ā, vs. short *a,* or ă), but it won't solve the problem with our game show partner when both the alphabet and the diacritical markings are different.

Fortunately, there is a common symbol system that can be used by linguists, phoneticians, speech-language pathologists, audiologists, teachers of the deaf, and any other professional who needs to characterize the pronunciation of speech: the **International Phonetic Alphabet (IPA)** (refer to Tables 1–1 and 1–2). Developed in 1886 and revised in 1993 and 1996, the IPA assigns a different symbol to each of the sounds of speech across all the world's languages. Each symbol corresponds to one, and only one, speech sound, or **phoneme.** For example, the *a* in *apple* is transcribed as /æ/, and the *a* in *bake* is transcribed as /eɪ/. Spelling of words can (and often will) be variable, but IPA transcription is consistent in its sound-symbol relationships.

Nevertheless, you, as a beginning student in phonetics, have spent many years reading and writing using the orthographic system of your language. Whether you realize it or not, you tend to view words in terms of alphabet letters rather than the

TABLE 1–1 INTERNATIONAL PHONETIC ALPHABET SYMBOLS: VOWELS AND DIPHTHONGS FOR MAINSTREAM AMERICAN ENGLISH[1]

Primary Orthographic Symbols	IPA Symbol	Key Words
ee	/i/	beet, meat
-i-	/ɪ/	bit, kiss
-e-	/ɛ/	bet, less
-a-	/æ/	bat, pass
-oo-	/u/	pool, too
-oo-	/ʊ/	book, could
-aw-	/ɔ/	saw, caught
-o-	/ɑ/	bond, odd
-ur-	/ɝ/	turn, earth, bird (stressed)
	/ɚ/	hamm<u>er</u>, und<u>er</u> (unstressed)
-u-	/ʌ/	up, come (stressed)
-u-	/ə/	el<u>e</u>phant, b<u>a</u>nan<u>a</u> (unstressed)
a-e	/eɪ/	<u>a</u>ble, m<u>a</u>de, m<u>ay</u> (stressed)
a-e	/e/	vibr<u>a</u>te, rot<u>a</u>te (unstressed)
oa	/oʊ/	code, own, boat (stressed)
oa	/o/	<u>o</u>bey, r<u>o</u>tation (unstressed)
i-e	/aɪ/	kite, ice, my
ou	/aʊ/	out, loud
oi	/ɔi/	coin, boy, oil

[1] Vowel symbols that are more characteristic of regional and cultural dialects will be introduced later in this book.

TABLE 1–2 INTERNATIONAL PHONETIC ALPHABET SYMBOLS: CONSONANTS FOR
MAINSTREAM AMERICAN ENGLISH

Primary Orthographic Symbols	IPA Symbols	Key Words
p	/p/	pie, stopped, sip
b	/b/	boy, baby, cub
t	/t/	top, later, seat
d	/d/	down, ladder, red
k	/k/	come, baker, book
g	/g/	go, bigger, log
f	/f/	four, offer, calf
v	/v/	vine, over, believe
th	/θ/	thorn, nothing, earth
th	/ð/	them, bother, breathe
s	/s/	see, bicycle, ice
z	/z/	zoo, buzzer, eyes
sh	/ʃ/	shoe, mushroom, dish
zh	/ʒ/	measure, beige
h	/h/	hide, behind
ch	/tʃ/	chair, matches, such
j	/dʒ/	jump, angel, fudge
w	/w/	we, awake
y	/j/	yes, bayou
l	/l/	listen, hollow, fill
r	/ɹ/	rain, arrange, car
m	/m/	me, omen, home
n	/n/	new, owner, pan
ng	/ŋ/	sing, singer

actual phonemes perceived. Consequently, you must learn to disregard what you know about spelling in order to master phonetics. In the next section, we will present a variety of examples to help you understand the importance of listening for phonemes, rather than visualizing word spellings. In addition, there are preparatory listening exercises in Chapter 1 of the workbook that will help you develop your listening skills.

ALPHABETIC LETTERS, SPEECH SOUNDS, AND THE INTERNATIONAL PHONETIC ALPHABET

WORD ORIGINS

The difference between the spelling of words and their pronunciation results from a variety of factors. As spoken language grows, it changes, but written language is slower to follow. Our English language originated from a variety of sources across Europe. These origins included Germanic dialects, Scandinavian languages (northern Europe), French, and romance languages (southern Europe), as well as classic Greek and Latin. Thus, two words can contain the same speech sound/phoneme but vary in their spelling as a result of their origin. For example, the first phoneme in the words *fan* and *phone* is the same (IPA transcription: /f/), but the spelling (*ph* or *f*) differs. The *ph* spelling is most likely indicative of the word's Greek origin, whereas the *f* spelling is indicative of Middle English and Latin origins.

We have also borrowed words from other languages, sometimes resulting in a great difference in spelling and the actual phonemes/pronunciation of a word. This is particularly obvious in words that English has borrowed from French. For example, *coup d'état* (or its shortened form, *coup*) is frequently heard in English. But suppose you pronounced it according to its English spelling (*koopdeetat* or *koop*). At best, no one would know what you were talking about. At worst, you would be the source of great amusement to all those who know the actual pronunciation, *koodaytah* ([k u d e t ɑ], using the IPA). It is this actual pronunciation, not spelling, that you must learn to focus on and transcribe, using the IPA.

INCONSISTENCIES IN THE ENGLISH ORTHOGRAPHIC SYSTEM

A major problem of orthography is that the Roman alphabet does not contain enough symbols to represent all the different English phonemes that you will learn to listen for. We have only 26 alphabet letters to represent 43 basic phonemes. You learned in elementary school that there are five vowels: *a, e, i, o,* and *u* (and sometimes *y*). Actually, there are 18 different vowel and diphthong phonemes in English and 25 different consonant phonemes (as opposed to the 21 orthographic letters). Some phonemes have no specific letter to represent them (e.g., the medial consonant in *lei̲sure* and *plea̲sure*). Still others require a combination of letters to stand for the single phoneme they represent (e.g., the initial sound in *sh̲oe* and *sh̲are* or those in *ch̲in* and *ch̲air*. Using the IPA, you will have one symbol for each of these phonemes: /ʃ/ for *sh* and /tʃ/ for *ch*. (These letter combinations are also known as **digraphs.**)

Next, we will demonstrate the need to focus on listening to speech sounds, rather than thinking of spelling, by considering how the same spelling does not equate to the same phonemes in different words. The words *chorus* and *choke* both begin with the same orthographic symbols, *ch*. However, the initial phonemes in these words are different (IPA: /k/ and /tʃ/. Similar examples are found in words such as *pressure* and *pressing*. The middle consonant phoneme is spelled as *ss* in each word, but they actually represent two different phonemes, *sh* (IPA: /ʃ/) and *s* (IPA: /s/).

On the other hand, spelling may differ even though the same phoneme is contained in two words. An illustration is in the words *sugar* and *shoe;* both start with the phoneme /ʃ/, but their spelling of that speech sound differs. Similarly, the sound of *f* (IPA: /f/) can be spelled in a variety of ways (e.g., *far, phantom, different,* and *cough*).

English spelling also includes letters for which there is no corresponding phoneme. In the word *knife,* for example, there are really only three phonemes (IPA: /n aɪ f/), but the spelling consists of five letters. If you look at the word *honest,* there are six orthographic letters, but there are only five phonemes (IPA: /ɑ n ə s t/

because the letter *h* is silent). The same principle applies to the word *house,* but a different letter is involved. The five letters in the word actually correspond to only three phonemes: /h aʊ s/. This time the *h* does symbolize a phoneme, but there is only one vowel (symbolized by two orthographic letters), and the *e* is silent.

The orthographic system for vowels also provides excellent (and often frustrating) examples of how the same orthographic letter does not necessarily represent the same phoneme in different words. Remember our example from the teacher of ESL students? Consider the orthographic symbol *o.* We use this letter to represent a number of different vowel phonemes, for example, *ton, top, told, tomb,* and *woman* (IPA symbols: /ʌ ɑ oʊ u ʊ/. Table 1–3 (Calvert, 1992) gives a quantitative picture of how variable the correspondence between spelling and pronunciation of vowels can be. With the IPA, each different vowel pronunciation has its own unique symbol, eliminating confusion.

For most Americans, these inconsistencies and irregularities are manageable obstacles to be overcome in learning to read and spell. This is not necessarily the case for children with reading disabilities or communication disorders. Furthermore, nonnative English speakers' mispronunciations are often related to the irregularities between orthographic spelling and the actual pronunciation of a word. Again, your key task in learning phonetics will be to listen for each sound and associate it

TABLE 1–3 PERCENTAGE OF TIMES EACH OF 19 ALPHABET SPELLINGS REPRESENTS THE DESIGNATED VOWEL SOUNDS IN 7500 COMMON WORDS

Orthographic Symbol	Word	Alphabet-Sound Agreement	Orthographic Symbol	Word	Alphabet-Sound Agreement
a-e	gave	100%	-a-	cat	83%
				table	13%
u-e	cute	100%			
			-u-	cup	73%
aw	law	100%		unite	24%
i-e	kite	99%	ea	meat	74%
				head	24%
oi	boil	99%			
oa	boat	98%	-e-	bet	70%
ee	beet	96%		be	30%
			ou	out	60%
-i-	pin	91%		rough	35%
	child	9%			
			oo	boot	59%
ai	bait	90%		cook	41%
au	caught	88%	-o-	top	53%
				told	40%
			ow	low	52%
				cow	48%
			o-e	home	34%
				come	66%

with its IPA symbol. Thinking about a word's spelling will not help, and more likely will hinder, your growth in this process.

BASIC TERMS AND DEFINITIONS
PHONETICS AND RELATED CONCEPTS

Phonetics, the focus of this textbook, is defined most simply as the study of speech sounds of spoken language. Within this broad definition, a number of subtypes or branches are important to the student of phonetics. In particular, we will emphasize **physiologic phonetics** and **acoustic phonetics** to build understanding of the English language sound system. Researchers in physiologic phonetics attempt to analyze speech sounds in terms of the anatomic and physiologic concepts involved. Thus, studies in physiologic phonetics would focus on the interaction of physical structures, muscles, and movements involved in producing speech sounds. For the acoustic phonetician, the focus is directed toward the acoustic properties of speech sounds, that is, the frequency and intensity of the actual sounds heard. Studies in acoustic phonetics might include investigating how different alterations of a speech signal affect the listener's ability to understand what was said.

We have noted that speech sounds, or phonemes, are the focus of study in phonetics. However, the definition of a phoneme is more complex than just "speech sound." In fact, each phoneme is actually a group of sounds, or **allophones.** Each time we produce a speech sound, we produce it in a slightly different way. As long as the formation and its acoustic result are consistent enough, we will hear each allophone as a representative of that specific phoneme class. For example, try saying the word *cap* in these two different ways. First, open your lips as you finish the word, so that lip closure for /p/ is followed by release of air. Next, say the word again, but keep your lips closed. You just produced two allophones of /p/, the aspirated (air released) and the unaspirated (air not released). Despite that small difference in air release, you still hear the last sound in both words as /p/. The same is true of other phonemes.

We will perceive allophonic variations of a particular phoneme as being that phoneme, only as long as certain requirements are met. For example, if you say *cap* and then *cat,* you hear two different phonemes at the end of the words. It does not matter whether you release the air or not; the places where the sounds are made differ: /p/ is made with the lips, and /t/ is made with the tongue tip and alveolar ridge. Requirements to hear an allophone as the phoneme /p/ include lip closure; tongue tip–alveolar ridge closure produces a different phoneme. Finally, a word that varies only by allophones (e.g., the two ways of saying /p/ in *cap*) will still be heard as two versions of the same word. Changing the phoneme /p/ to /t/ in *cap* and *cat,* however, results in a difference in meaning; that is, the phoneme change means that you hear two different words.

IPA transcription of words may or may not reflect allophonic variation. **Broad transcription** (also known as **phonemic transcription**) does not reflect allophonic variation and is contained in soliduses (/ /). If you wished to reflect the difference between our two allophones of /p/ (previous example), you would have to use **narrow transcription** (also known as **phonetic transcription**).

Phonetic transcription, enclosed in brackets ([   ]), includes **diacritic markings** to reflect allophonic differences. Thus, a phonemic transcription of *cap* (both aspirated and unaspirated) would be /k æ p/. A phonetic, or narrow, transcription would have to represent each word separately and use diacritical markings indicative of aspiration: [k æ p^h] (aspirated/air released) and [k æ p˺] (air not released).

PHONOLOGY AND MEANING

There is more to understanding phonemes than just how they are formed and perceived. Phonetics is related to another area of study, **phonology.** Whereas phoneticians focus on formation and acoustic characteristics of phonemes, phonologists are interested in how phonemes can be combined to transmit meaning. This is not as simple as it might sound. In English, some phoneme combinations are not possible or typical. For example, the phoneme /ŋ/ (as in *hang*) cannot initiate words in English. English allows word-beginning consonant clusters or blends of up to three sounds (e.g., *splash*) but does not permit four-consonant blends to initiate a word. The Russian word for *hello* (transliterated as *sdrastvweetyeh*) seems hard to pronounce for English speakers because it combines consonant phonemes in ways not permitted in English.

Developmental phonology is the study of how children acquire the sound system of their language. Early in development, children often omit final consonants in words. Because final consonants are important in signaling meaning in English, the child must eventually learn to "close" words with them. If the child fails to do so in a timely manner, he or she is said to have a **phonological disorder.**

Phonemes signal meaning within the context of **morphemes.** Morphemes are the smallest meaningful units of language. A morpheme may consist of one or more phonemes or a word. A word may contain more than one morpheme. The word *view* is composed of one morpheme; it cannot be broken down further and still retain its meaning. However, if we add the phoneme /s/, we change the meaning: *views* means "more than one view" and contains two morphemes (*view* + *s*). If we then add the prefix *pre-*, we have created a word with three morphemes (*pre-* + *view* + *s,* or *previews*). The meaningful words (one morpheme each) *cat* and *cap* give us an example of how phonemes differentiate meaning within the context of morphemes. *Cat* and *cap* differ in their final phonemes, /t/ and /p/. It is that simple difference in phonemes that tells us whether someone is talking about a furry feline or a hat.

You will learn to recognize and transcribe the phonemes of English primarily within the context of words as you progress through this book and its accompanying workbook. This puts these physiological and acoustic units into their language role: to signal differences in meaning. We can better understand how oral language can be made clear and understandable by learning about phonemes and transcribing them as units that differentiate meaning.

REVIEW VOCABULARY

acoustic phonetics   study of acoustic features of speech and their relationship to speech production and speech perception.

acoustics   branch of physics concerned with the physical properties of sound.

allophone   examples of variations within a phoneme class; heard as one/same phoneme.

broad transcription   in IPA, transcribing in phoneme symbols only, without modifying (diacritical) markings to indicate allophonic or other phonetic differences; uses /   /.

developmental phonology   study of child's acquisition of speech sounds and the rules governing their usage.

diacritic markings   symbols used to modify alphabet letters or phonetic symbols to indicate differences in pronunciation.

digraph   combination of alphabetic symbols that represent one phoneme.

International Phonetic Alphabet (IPA)   a symbol system in which any phoneme used in a language (or across languages) has one, and only one, symbol.

narrow transcription   in IPA, transcribing in phoneme symbols plus modifying markings to indicate variations in pronunciation; uses [   ].

morpheme   smallest unit of phonological form(s) that signals a difference in meaning.

orthography   commonly accepted spelling using alphabet symbols.

phoneme   an abstract class of speech sounds containing common elements and influencing the meaning of speech.

phonemic transcription   identical to broad transcription.

phonetic transcription   identical to narrow transcription.

phonetics   science devoted to the study of speech sounds.

phonological disorder   failure to master the sound system rules characteristic of a particular language.

phonology   area of linguistic study focused on speech sounds and the combination of those sounds to transmit meaning.

physiologic phonetics   study of interactions of physical structures, muscles, and movements in producing speech sounds.

transliteration   selecting alphabet letters to represent speech sounds.

EXERCISES

As you learned in this chapter, the relationship between phonemes and their orthographic representation can be highly variable. The following exercises are designed to help you develop your listening skills and decrease your reliance on visual orthographic symbols. In each exercise, remember to focus on phonemes, not letters.

Consonant Exercises

1. Orthographic consonant digraphs use two letters to stand for one phoneme. In the following words, circle each consonant digraph that actually is heard as a single phoneme.

thorn   fresh   father   ledge   chain   long
wish   phony   think   ring   wreath   then

2. Two or more orthographic letters may be used to represent a single consonant phoneme. In the following words, circle the two consecutive consonants that represent a single consonant phoneme.

supper   passing   petting   lotto   berry   willing
shrugged   mall   tripped   scuff

3. Orthography can include letters for which there is no corresponding phoneme (e.g., silent letters). In the following words, circle the letters that are silent/have no corresponding phoneme.

limb   know   mnemonic   psychiatry   gnash
knew   psalm   paradigm   autumn

4. Alphabetic letters do not always have a consistent one-to-one relationship with phonemes. In the following word lists, circle the two words that contain a different phoneme than the other four, even though the spelling is the same.

a.   chain   choose   chorus   cheek   chill   chic
b.   sugar   treasure   insured   conscience   assure   lose

5. This time, circle all the words that contain the same phoneme, regardless of spelling/letters. Then, using Table 1–2, determine which IPA symbol represents the common sound.

a.	zinc	tans	Susan	leisure	fuzzy	pats	/ /
b.	mission	oceanic	anchored	sheep	chance	tissue	/ /
c.	regal	singe	jump	badge	gyp	single	/ /
d.	island	box	sounds	confusion	pace	mercy	/ /
e.	yes	fuse	four	canyon	onion	fussy	/ /
f.	whose	hang	honesty	leather	behind	hole	/ /
g.	rough	funny	phoneme	of	oven	graph	/ /
h.	grow	high	lozenge	again	begin	pig	/ /

Vowel Exercises

6. In orthographics, two letters can actually stand for only one vowel phoneme. In the following words, circle the two letters that correspond to only one phoneme.

boat   outer   coupe   maid   boast   round
moon   oiled   pain   division   sooner   bait

7. Orthographics can also contain letters for which there is no corresponding vowel phoneme. In the following words, circle the letters that are silent.

lode   caged   entered   cave   matched   done

8. Spelling does not necessarily correspond to the actual vowel represented. In each of the following lists of similarly spelled words, circle the word(s)

that have a different vowel phoneme, even though all the words are spelled alike.

a.   gown   hollow   coward   crow   frown
b.   shoe   poet   hoed   doe

9. In contrast to the examples in #8, words can share the same vowel but differ greatly in spelling. For the following word lists, circle the words that have the same vowel phoneme. Then, using Table 1–1, find the IPA symbol representing that vowel.

a.   train   feign   deceive   lane   pack   paper   /   /
b.   beak   seat   peas   rein   meet   tread   /   /
c.   graph   knot   vat   manic   pane   trash   /   /
d.   took   soup   flew   ruse   plume   foot   /   /
e.   pad   possible   comb   palm   bond   soggy   /   /
f.   pun   son   under   trouble   coupe   bond   /   /
g.   might   insist   bitters   pitch   inside   piece   /   /
h.   count   good   should   cook   full   sloop   /   /

CHAPTER 2

THE SPEECH PRODUCTION MECHANISM AND PROCESSES

THE SPEECH MECHANISM: SUPRAGLOTTAL STRUCTURES
THE LARYNX AND SUBGLOTTAL STRUCTURES
SPEECH PROCESSES AND ASSOCIATED STRUCTURES
REVIEW VOCABULARY
EXERCISES

Among the creatures of Earth, only humans have achieved speech. All species of animals communicate, many through vocalizations, but none have approached the complexity and sophistication of our oral language. Yet the body parts we use to produce speech do not appear to be vastly different from those of other animals that also have teeth, tongues, and palates. Like other species, we use these oral structures regularly for basic biological functions such as breathing and eating. However, we know that a healthy human infant has an innate potential to communicate orally. Research tells us that humans have some unique neurological and structural characteristics that allow us to use these body parts for speech production in addition to their basic, vegetative function.

Speech is actually the end product of four processes or actions that occur simultaneously and cooperatively: respiration, phonation, resonation, and articulation. It is very important to understand the implications of the terms *simultaneously* and *cooperatively.* Speaking is not a linear sequence of events that begins with the lungs and ends with the listener's ear. The act of speaking requires continuous, overlapping action as well as feedback adjustments across all the systems involved. In order to understand the speech processes, we begin with a description of the basic structures involved in speech production.

THE SPEECH MECHANISM: SUPRAGLOTTAL STRUCTURES

As we review the structures of the speech mechanism, we will cover vegetative (biological) function, speech functions, and terms commonly associated with each stucture. Although we will discuss the structures of the speech mechanism separately, remember that all these structures function synergistically to produce speech. To emphasize the interaction, we have grouped the structures according to location and function.

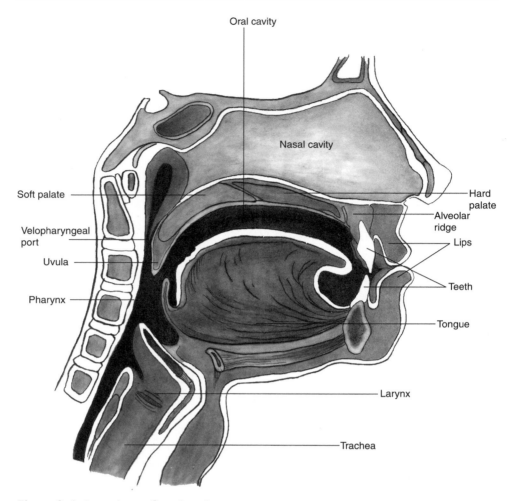

Figure 2–1 *Sagittal view of speech mechanism.*

THE SUPRALARYNGEAL STRUCTURES

The supralaryngeal structures refer to those parts of the speech mechanism located above the level of the larynx. Each of these structures is contained in one of three cavities or spaces: **oral, nasal,** or **pharyngeal.** The **pharyngeal cavity,** or **pharynx,** extends from the opening of the larynx to the posterior boundaries of the **oral cavity** (mouth) and **nasal cavity** (nose) (see Figure 2–1). Positioning and movements of the structures in these cavities shape the outgoing airstream into the vowels and consonants we recognize as speech.

ORAL CAVITY   The lips are the external boundary of the oral cavity. They are actually a complex of muscles and other tissues. For vegetative functions, they help receive and contain food and fluids in the oral cavity. In speech, they perform a variety of actions. For vowels, lip position can range from rounded to neutral to spread. These changes in shape contribute to the resonant pattern that characterizes different vowels. Several consonants are classified as **labial** (involving the lips). Some of these consonants are **bilabial** (both lips used), such as /b/, and others are

labiodental (lips and teeth used), such as /v/. In most speakers, the lower lip is more mobile in rapid, connected speech.

TEETH   The role of the teeth for life support is an obvious one: cutting and grinding food. Their speech role is primarily passive but nonetheless important. In English, two consonants are classified as **dental** or **interdental** (involving the teeth): the /θ/ in *thorn* and the /ð/ in *them*. However, production of a number of consonants such as /s/ and /z/ requires that the back sides of the tongue be sealed against the back teeth (molars) to direct the airstream appropriately. Otherwise, air may escape laterally, resulting in a distortion of the sound(s). Loss of the central **incisors** (front teeth) between ages 5 and 7 results in many children having a **lisp** (/s/) problem. The problem disappears when the permanent incisors grow in fully.

ALVEOLAR RIDGE   In both the **maxilla** (upper jaw) and **mandible** (lower jaw), the teeth are contained in the **alveolar ridge** (alveolar processes, more commonly known as the "gum ridges"). Biologically, the alveolar ridge serves as an important surface for tongue contact in the act of swallowing. In speech, many consonants involve tongue contact with, or placement near, the upper alveolar ridge, which is found behind the maxillary incisors and cuspid teeth. Alveolar consonants such as /t/, /s/, and /l/, to name just a few, involve the maxillary alveolar ridge. In addition, the alveolar ridge, along with the anterior palate, serves as a "reference point" for the tongue in front vowel formation.

HARD PALATE   The hard **palate** is composed of bony tissue and covered by the mucous membrane. It divides the oral and nasal cavities, forming the roof of the oral cavity and the floor of the nasal cavity. For life-sustaining purposes, the palate helps contain food in the oral cavity and provides a hard upper surface for swallowing. It is involved in both vowel and consonant production for speech. For vowels, it plays a role in oral cavity shaping. Several consonants are considered palatal: /ʃ/, /ʒ/, /tʃ/, /dʒ/, /r/, and /j/. All require the tongue to be positioned near, or to move in relation to, the palate.

SOFT PALATE   Posterior to the hard palate, the **velum** or **soft palate** forms the roof of the mouth. It is composed of muscle and connective tissue and is covered by a continuation of the mucous membrane of the hard palate. Biologically, its action is necessary to prevent foods and fluid from entering the nasal cavity. Opening and closing of the **velopharyngeal port** (aperture/opening that connects the nasal and oral cavity) require participation of the velum. Its muscular composition makes it highly flexible and important for speech function. By helping to close the velopharyngeal port, the velum helps direct the breath stream to the oral cavity for articulation of oral resonant phonemes, especially vowels. Relaxation of the velum opens the velopharyngeal port and is necessary to produce the three nasal consonant phonemes /m/, /n/, and /ŋ/. Consonants involving tongue contact with the velum, /k/, /g/, and /ŋ/, are referred to as **velar** consonants.

TONGUE   The tongue (adjective, **lingual-/-lingua**) is composed of muscle and connective tissue and covered by the mucous membrane. It is of extreme importance for both biological purposes and speech. Its role in life functions is crucial: directing food to the back of the oral cavity in swallowing. Highly flexible and mobile, the tongue can shape the oral cavity almost infinitely. It arises from the floor of

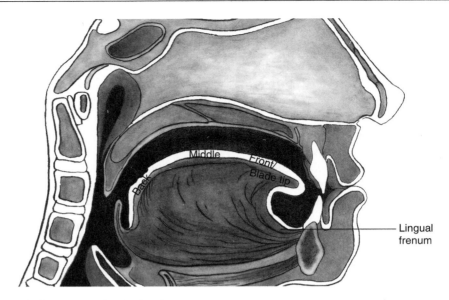

Figure 2–2 *Tongue surface landmarks.*

the oral cavity and is dually controlled by both intrinsic (within the tongue) and extrinsic (connecting the tongue to other structures) muscles. To understand the specific role of the tongue in vowel and consonant production, you need to be familiar with various tongue landmarks. The tongue itself has a root, apex, dorsum, septum, and frenum. The root is the posterior portion, connecting to the hyoid bone and the epiglottis. The anterior end of the tongue is its **apex,** and the superior (upper) surface, the **dorsum.** The **lingual septum** is actually a midline structure of connective tissue. The front tongue undersurface is connected to the mandible by the **lingual frenum.** In describing speech articulation, we refer to various landmarks on the tongue surface: **back, middle, front/blade,** and **tip** (see Figure 2–2). Consonants such as /s/ and /t/ involve the tip, whereas /k/ and /g/ involve the back. In producing consonants and vowels, the tongue shape can vary from broad to narrow, flat to curled, and whole tongue positioning to differential positioning of tongue segments. All the vowels and most of the consonants require tongue action. Only /m/, /p/, /b/, /f/, and /v/ do not.

MANDIBLE   The mandible, or lower jaw, plays both an active and a passive role in articulation of speech sounds. It forms the base for the tongue and houses the mandibular teeth. Biologically, its rotary action is necessary for chewing. For speech, the mandible can be raised or lowered by varying degrees, contributing to changes in vowel articulation.

NASAL CAVITY   The nasal cavity lies directly superior to the oral cavity. Horizontally, it extends from the external nares (nostrils) to the posterior pharyngeal wall. Vertically, it is bounded by the base of the skull and the palate and velum. Its primary purpose is to receive inhaled air, filter it, warm it, and direct it toward the trachea (windpipe). With its soft, moist lining, it contributes to the distinctive resonance characteristics of the cavity. The nasal cavity participates in speech resonance with either closure or opening of the velopharyngeal port. It is always open anteriorly, at the nostrils, unless you have a cold or other infection. Even if the velopharyngeal port is closed, the nasal cavity resonates the vibrating airstream from the larynx. In this case, the combined resonation of oral and nasal air produces an individual speaker's distinctive voice quality. Production of /m/, /n/, and /ŋ/ requires closure somewhere in the oral cavity combined with opening of the velopharyngeal port (lowering the velum). This allows the nasal cavity to serve as the primary resonator.

PHARYNGEAL CAVITY   Anatomically, the pharynx (pharyngeal cavity) extends from the posterior portion of the nasal cavity downward past the back of the oral cavity to (but not including) the larynx (see Figure 2–1). Biological functions include (1) receiving food from swallowing and moving it toward the esophagus and stomach and (2) channeling air from respiration between the nose and mouth, trachea and lungs. A vertical tube, the pharynx actually can be subdivided into three parts: the nasopharynx (continuation of the nasal cavity), the oropharynx (continuation of the oral cavity), and the laryngopharynx (just above the larynx). For speech production, the pharynx acts as a resonating chamber for the voice. (Although some languages use the pharynx for consonant articulation, English is not one of them.) The primary pharyngeal alteration is velopharyngeal closure that both directs the voice into the oral cavity and reduces the length of the pharyngeal tube (by closing off the nasopharynx). Pharyngeal circumference can also be changed by constriction or relaxation of the muscular pharyngeal walls. Such changes alter the resonating characteristics of the pharynx and, consequently, the sound of the human voice.

THE LARYNX AND SUBGLOTTAL STRUCTURES

The **larynx** is composed of cartilage and muscle. It sits on top of, and is connected to, the trachea (see Figure 2–3A, B). Its most crucial life support function is protection of the lungs by preventing food particles and fluids from entering the trachea. Any food materials that enter the larynx are expelled by coughing. Other vegetative functions include closing the trachea so that air is held in the chest (**thoracic**) cavity. This frees the muscles such as the pectoralis major from respiration and allows them to participate in important tasks such as heavy lifting.

The larynx (adjective, **laryngo-/-laryngeal**) is suspended from the **hyoid bone** by a complex of muscles and ligaments and lies posterior and slightly inferior to the tongue root. It contains the **vocal folds** necessary for **phonation** (vocal fold vibration). The vocal folds are actually "shelves" of muscles and connective tissue, lined with mucous membrane. The space between the vocal folds is referred to as the **glottis**, and sometimes laryngeal structures are referred to as **subglottal** or **supraglottal**, depending on their spatial relationship with the vocal fold opening. The vocal folds are anchored to the inner surface of the large **thyroid cartilage** anteriorly. Posteriorly, the folds attach to the movable **arytenoid cartilages.** These cartilages allow the vocal folds to be **abducted** (positioned apart) or **adducted** (positioned together, or **approximated**) (see Figure 2–4). Inferiorly, the **cricoid cartilage** forms the base of the larynx and rests atop the trachea. In summary, then, the structures important to laryngeal function are cricoid cartilage, paired arytenoid cartilages, thyroid cartilage, hyoid bone, and vocal folds.

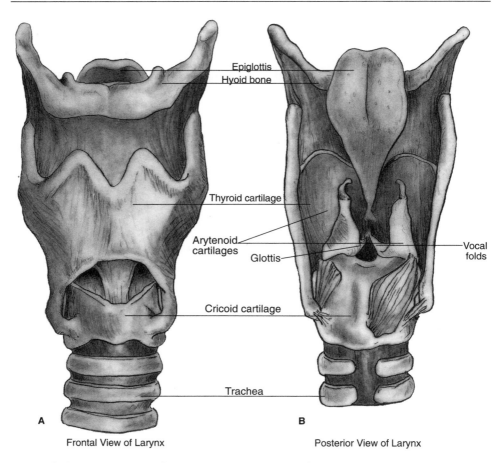

Epiglottis
Hyoid bone
Thyroid cartilage
Arytenoid cartilages
Glottis
Vocal folds
Cricoid cartilage
Trachea

A   B
Frontal View of Larynx   Posterior View of Larynx

Figure 2–3 *(A) Frontal view of the larynx. (B) Posterior view of the larynx.*

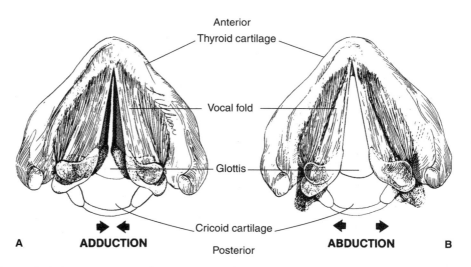

Anterior
Thyroid cartilage
Vocal fold
Glottis
Cricoid cartilage
Posterior

A   **ADDUCTION**   **ABDUCTION**   B

Figure 2–4 *(A) Superior view of the larynx: vocal fold adduction. (B) Superior view of the larynx: vocal fold abduction.*

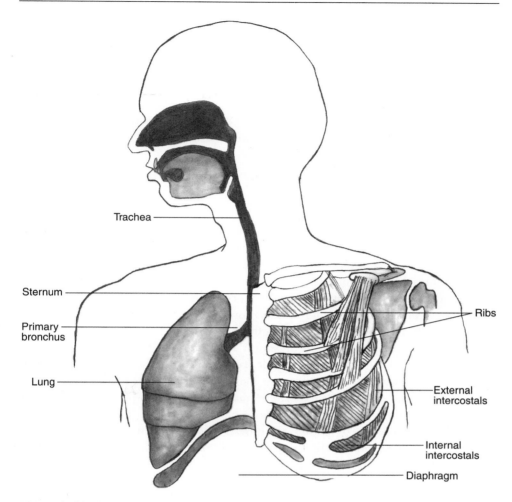

Figure 2–5 *Sublaryngeal structures.*

Phonemes that are produced with vocal fold vibration (vocal folds adducted) are referred to as **voiced** sounds; those produced with the vocal folds abducted are **voiceless.** All American English vowels and the majority of consonants are voiced.

Sublaryngeal structures are the organs of respiration that provide the breath stream necessary for speech production (see Figure 2–5). The **trachea** is immediately below (and attached to) the cricoid cartilage. It is actually a tube of cartilaginous rings and other connective tissue that descends in front of the esophagus and bifurcates (divides in half) into two primary **bronchi.** The paired bronchi enter the lungs and continue to bifurcate into smaller **bronchioles.** Ultimately, the bronchioles terminate in the **alveolar ducts,** which lead to the **alveolar sacs.** The **alveoli** are contained in the walls of the alveolar sacs and serve as the site for the exchange of oxygen and carbon dioxide. Other sublaryngeal structures necessary for life support and speech include the **rib cage, diaphragm,** and other muscles of respiration.

SPEECH PROCESSES AND ASSOCIATED STRUCTURES

Now that you are familiar with the structures involved in the speech process, we will discuss their integrated roles in speech production. The resulting, overlapping processes of respiration, phonation, resonation, and articulation together are responsible for the variety of sounds we use to transmit as oral language. Coordination of these processes requires complex interaction, feedback, and adjustments, mediated by the nervous system (brain, cranial nerves, and spinal cord).

RESPIRATION

Human oral communication requires some type of air source for its occurrence. That source is provided by the process of respiration. Respiration is accomplished by a complex interaction of respiratory structures and muscles. The structures involved in respiration, as we noted earlier, include the lungs, bronchi, bronchioles, alveoli, and trachea. The muscles involved in respiration primarily include the diaphragm and the external and internal **intercostal muscles** (see Figure 2–5). However, respiration for speech requires more than just structures and muscle activity, as you will discover in the next section.

Whether breathing for speech or simply breathing quietly (life support), you inhale (bring air into the lungs) and exhale (release air from the lungs). Oxygen and carbon dioxide exchange occurs in the lungs each time you inhale and exhale, whether you speak or not. The exhalation phase of respiration provides the flow of breath for speech.

Inhalation consists of taking air into the lungs. Contraction of the diaphragm causes expansion of the thoracic cavity space. Co-occurring upward and outward rib cage movement due to the action of the thoracic and neck muscles also expands this space. The elastic properties of the lungs allow them to expand. Oxygen and carbon dioxide exchange occurs in the alveoli of the lungs. **Exhalation** (which provides the **egressive,** or outgoing, airstream for speech) is achieved by a combination of these factors: (1) gravity, (2) elastic properties of cartilage and lung tissue, and (3) relaxation of the muscles of inhalation. In addition, for speech and heavy breathing, there is progressive contraction of muscles of exhalation.

In normal breathing, the relative duration of inhalation and exhalation is about the same. But in speaking, the duration of exhalation in a single respiratory cycle is usually about 10 times longer than that of inhalation. Practiced speakers may actually have their exhalation phase last 50 times longer than inhalation. Despite differences in inhalatory and exhalatory cycle length for life support and speech, the actual amount of air exchanged is about the same, regardless of purpose. The extended duration of exhalation for speech reflects extremely efficient control of the breath stream. This efficiency results from the synergistic functioning of the respiratory muscles, larynx, and articulatory mechanisms. Changes in the larynx and articulatory system cause adjustments in the exhalation process. This degree of control takes time to master; consider how babies may cry and become out of breath but how a trained singer can easily sustain a note for a long period.

PHONATION

Phonation, or voicing, is accomplished by the interruption of the outgoing air-stream by rapid rhythmic closing and opening of the glottis with the vocal folds. The vocal folds are steadily but lightly approximated (together) when the arytenoid cartilages are adducted by muscle action. This degree of closing allows the folds to be parted by accumulated subglottal air pressure coming from the lungs. The folds then reapproximate from the combined effects of muscular tension and aero-dynamic effect. For phonation to occur, subglottal pressure must be sufficient to overcome both supraglottal air pressure and the glottal resistance or tension of the vocal folds. The actual process follows this rhythmic cycle:

1. Closing of the glottis
2. Increasing of air pressure beneath the glottis
3. Bursting apart of the folds from air pressure with release of a "puff" of compressed breath
4. Reclosing of the folds under constant muscle tension, with temporarily decreased subglottal air pressure drawing or "sucking" the folds back together

Air pressure beneath the glottis increases as air continues to flow from the lungs and trachea. Consequently, the cycle is repeated many times per second. The actual opening and closing of the folds is not a simple open and shut process. As previously noted, the vocal folds are actually muscular tissue shelves with vertical depth. Consequently, in each phonatory cycle, the folds open from bottom to top and from posterior to anterior. In closing, the inferior part of the folds closes before the superior part, and horizontal closure proceeds from anterior to posterior. When seen using high-speed photography, the motion of the folds actually appears wavelike. Each complete opening and closing of the glottis constitutes one cycle.

The rate of release of these puffs of air determines the **fundamental frequency,** or F_0 of a speaker's voice. Fundamental frequency varies, affected by age, gender, and voluntary control. For men, the average fundamental frequency of vocal fold vibration is 125 **hertz** (Hz, or cycles per second). The average fundamental frequency for women is faster, about 220 Hz. Not surprisingly, the fundamental frequency of infants' and children's voices is even faster. A faster F_0 is heard as a higher **pitch,** whereas a slower F_0 characterizes lower pitch.

Interaction of the lungs and the larynx is required for changes in fundamental frequency. Size and mass of the vocal folds determine the range of frequencies possible for a given speaker. You can change F_0 through a combination of alterations of (1) vocal fold tension and (2) subglottal air pressure. Higher or rising F_0 is associated with greater vocal fold tension and higher subglottal air pressure. A drop in F_0, conversely, is associated with a reduction in vocal fold tension and, especially, lower subglottal pressure. When you are conversing (rapid connected speech), your fundamental frequency will vary constantly according to these two factors of vocal fold tension and subglottal air pressure. That variation is perceived as changes in intonation of your voice.

More than fundamental frequency is produced by the rapid opening and closing of the glottis. As we noted, the movement of the folds is complex, and the folds actually open more slowly than they close. Consequently, a complex harmonic sound is produced by the opening and closing of the vocal folds. This secondary complex harmonic signal is composed of **harmonics** or overtones of the fundamental frequency. Thus, the sound that emerges is complex, more of a buzz. It is not recognizable as the human voice. Instead, it must pass through the resonatory system to develop those characteristics.

Intensity of voice, heard by listeners as loudness, results from an interaction of vocal fold characteristics and subglottal and supraglottal pressure. Greater loudness results from (1) increased subglottal pressure; (2) vocal fold control that allows rapid, firm, longer closure; and (3) expansion of the vocal tract for reduced supraglottal pressure. The opposite adjustments produce a more quiet voice intensity. Thus, a speaker whose voice is too soft can learn how to change respiration, phonation, and resonation to develop a louder voice.

In summary, vocal fold vibration is affected not only by the function of laryngeal structures but also by respiration (subglottal pressure) and resonation (supraglottal shaping and pressure). Feedback between and among these systems causes changes in their actions, resulting in the complex sound waveform that serves as the basis for speech.

Resonation

Resonation occurs as the vibrating airstream passes through the pharyngeal, oral, and nasal cavities. These cavities can be altered in size, shape, and coupling, or connections. The resonating cavities selectively amplify parts of the complex sound produced by phonation. The result is what you perceive as the distinctive sound of an individual's voice, also known as **voice quality.**

That quality of a person's voice is produced primarily by a combination of the person's habitual F_0 range blended with the overtones that are amplified (made louder) or subdued by resonation. The influences of resonation on voice quality include

1. The overall length of the vocal tract
2. The relative length of the oral, nasal, and pharyngeal cavities
3. Habitual muscle tensing (This can raise the larynx, which will change the size and shape of the pharynx.)
4. The size of the tongue in relation to the oral cavity
5. The moistness and softness of the cavity walls (Greater moistness and softness is associated with a lower, more "hollow"-sounding voice.)
6. The relative opening of the jaw and lips during speaking (Wider openings correspond to amplification of higher frequencies.)
7. Relative openness of the velopharyngeal port during production of vowels and oral resonant consonants (Greater opening will give a "nasal" quality to the voice.)

The low resonance pattern characteristic of the Disney cartoon character Goofy voice exemplifies the interaction of these factors. The low, hollow-sounding voice of this character is produced by tongue posture low and back (greater cavity space), small openings (lips, between resonating cavities), and soft, moist cavity walls. These adjustments amplify lower harmonics and are associated with the character's distinctive voice.

Overall, the process of resonation shapes and amplifies selected frequencies of the laryngeal tone. It does not occur in isolation but is affected by the nature of respiration, phonation, and articulation processes. It also plays a role in articulation, as you will see in the next section.

ARTICULATION

Articulation is defined as the shaping of the voiced or unvoiced breath stream to form the sounds of speech. The vowels and resonant consonants (/m/, /n/, /ŋ/, /l/, /r/, /w/, and /j/) are articulated primarily by adjustments in resonance. For example, the nasal consonants /m/, /n/, and /ŋ/ are all articulated with the velopharyngeal port open, or coupled to the pharynx. For /m/, the lips are closed (bilabial); for /n/, the tongue tip touches the alveolar ridge (lingua-alveolar). The fairly fixed position of the oral articulators, combined with the open velopharyngeal port, produces the distinctive resonance characteristics of nasal consonants. For /l/ and /r/ production, the voiced airstream flows through relatively fixed oral articulators, and the velopharyngeal port is closed. Additionally, the characteristic resonances of different vowels are produced by adjustments in the oral cavity.

In contrast, the remaining consonants are shaped by the action of the tongue, jaw, and lips. The velopharyngeal port is closed for articulation of these consonants. If airflow is constricted between maxillary incisors and lower lip, /f/ (unvoiced airstream) or /v/ (voiced airstream) results. This friction-like quality is also characteristic of nonresonant consonants produced with constriction in other parts of the oral cavity, for example, the alveolar ridge (/s/) and palate (/ʃ/). Another type of nonresonant consonant is produced when the outgoing airstream is suddenly stopped and (sometimes) released. Such closure with the lips produces the bilabial /p/ (unvoiced) and /b/ (voiced). Similarly, air is stopped between the tongue tip and the alveolar ridge for /t/ and /d/. Detailed descriptions of the articulatory process will be found in Chapters 3, 4, and 5.

Even this short discussion should make it clear that speech production is not a simple, one-step-at-a-time process, beginning with the lungs and ending with a stream of articulated speech sounds. The breath stream for speech, provided by the respiratory system, is constantly adjusting in response to the activity of the vocal folds, resonators, and articulators. Laryngeal changes in frequency of vibration characterize connected speech and also require reciprocal adjustments across systems. Precise timing between articulation and phonation is necessary to produce appropriate voicing for consonants. Upper airway pressure changes, resulting from movement of the articulators, require changes in the glottis and the respiratory system. If each process operated independently of each other, fluent speech would be impossible. It is the simultaneous and cooperative functioning of these systems and their structures that allows us to produce speech.

REVIEW VOCABULARY

abducted/abduction   structures drawn apart from the midline (e.g., when the vocal folds are abducted, the glottis is open).

adducted/adduction   structures drawn together toward the midline (e.g., when the vocal folds are adducted, the glottis is closed).

alveolar ridge   prominent ridge behind the maxillary incisors and the cuspid (canine) teeth.

alveoli   located in the alveolar sacs (termination of alveolar ducts) in the lungs; site of actual exchange of oxygen and carbon dioxide.

apex (tongue)   anterior end of the tongue.

approximated   degree of closeness of vocal folds.

articulation   shaping of outgoing breath stream into the sounds of speech.

arytenoid cartilages   small, pyramidal-shaped cartilages that rest on top of the posterior cricoid cartilage; form movable, posterior attachments for vocal folds.

bilabial   both lips.

blade (of tongue)   part of the dorsum of the tongue immediately behind the tip; also known as the front of the tongue.

bronchi (singular bronchus)   two primary divisions from the trachea that lead into the right and left lung.

bronchioles   smaller branches of the bronchi.

cricoid cartilage   ring-shaped base/most inferior cartilage of the larynx; arytenoid cartilages are positioned superiorly on its posterior expanded portion.

dental   referring to the teeth; (inter)dental consonants are produced with the tongue tip against or between the teeth.

diaphragm   primary muscle of inhalation; dome-shaped, separating the abdominal and thoracic cavities.

dorsum (tongue)   upper surface of tongue.

egressive   outgoing; refers to airstream in exhalation.

exhalation   expulsion of air from the lungs; provides outgoing airstream for speech; half of a respiratory cycle.

fundamental frequency (F_0)   in reference to voice, rate at which the glottis opens and closes; measured in Hz. During phonation; heard by listener as pitch of voice.

glottis   space between the vocal folds; may be open or closed; adjective, *glottal*.

harmonic   a sound that is harmonic has a systematic pattern of vibration that is repeated at regular time intervals.

harmonics   soundwave components, that, when added together, join to make a single complex motion.

hertz (Hz)   refers to frequency of vibration/number of vibratory cycles per second.

hyoid bone   bone that does not directly articulate (form a joint with) any other bone but is held in position by muscles and connective tissues; the larynx is suspended from it; prefix, *hyo-*.

incisors   eight teeth (four maxillary, four mandibular) used for cutting; two central incisors, two lateral incisors per jaw.

inhalation   drawing of air into the lungs, result of action of the diaphragm and elastic forces; half of a respiratory cycle.

intensity   with regard to vocal fold vibration, amount of displacement of folds; perceived as loudness.

intercostal muscles   muscles of respiration attached to ribs, involved in inhalation (external intercostals) and exhalation (internal intercostals).

interdental   referring to phoneme articulation involving teeth and tongue tip.

labial   referring to the lips.

labiodental   referring to the lips and teeth.

laryngo-/laryngeal   referring to the larynx.

lingual frenum   tissue connecting the front part of the tongue to the floor of the oral cavity/mandible.

lingual septum   internal midline structure of the tongue, composed of connective tissue.

lisp   problem articulating the phoneme /s/.

mandible   lower jaw; adjective, mandibular.

maxilla   upper jaw; adjective, maxillary.

nasal   referring to the nose or nasal cavity.

nasal cavity   the nose, bounded by the nostrils and pharynx (anterior-posterior) and the palate and base of the skull (inferior-superior).

oral   referring to the mouth or oral cavity.

oral cavity   the mouth, bounded by the lips and pharynx (anterior-posterior) and the mandible and palate (inferior-superior).

palate (hard)   refers to the hard, bony roof of the mouth, dividing the oral cavity from the nasal cavity; adjective, palatal.

pharyngeal   referring to the pharynx.

pharyngeal cavity (pharynx)   the throat, that part of the vocal tract bounded by the larynx and oral and nasal cavities. Three subdivisions: laryngopharynx, oropharynx, and nasopharynx.

phonation   vocal fold vibration, produced in the larynx.

pitch   the property of a sound that is determined by the frequency of vibration.

resonation   process of modifying a sound by passing it through a cavity of air.

rib cage   bony framework encasing the lungs; movement involved in respiration.

soft palate   see Velum.

subglottal structures   structures inferior to the glottis (e.g., cricoid cartilage and trachea).

sublaryngeal structures   portions of the speech tract lying inferior to the laryngeal structures; consist of lungs, bronchi, bronchioles, alveoli, and trachea. Also known as the respiratory system.

supraglottal structures   structures lying superior to the glottis (e.g., epiglottis and tongue).

thoracic   related to the thorax.

thorax   body cavity containing heart and lungs bounded by spinal column, ribcage, sternum, and diaphragm.

thyroid cartilage   largest cartilage in the larynx, its halves are closed anteriorly and open posteriorly; anterior attachment point for vocal folds.

tongue tip   most anterior point of tongue; used for articulation of many consonants.

trachea   windpipe, composed of cartilaginous rings, connecting the larynx with the bronchi and lungs.

velopharyngeal port   opening that connects the nasopharynx and the oropharynx.

velum   the soft muscular posterior third of the roof of the mouth, attached to the hard palate; can be raised or lowered; adjective, *velar*.

vocal folds   muscular shelves in the larynx, extending from the thyroid cartilage (anteriorly) to the arytenoid cartilages (posteriorly).

voice quality   the distinctive sound resulting from a combination of habitual range of fundamental frequency, blended with overtones amplified or subdued through resonation.

voiced/voiceless   refers to the presence/absence of vocal fold vibration. Voiced sounds are produced with vocal fold vibration; voiceless sounds are produced without vocal fold vibration.

EXERCISES

1. List the structure(s) associated with the following terms:
   a. bilabial _____*lips*_____   e. pharyngeal _____*pharynx*_____
   b. glottal _____*vocal folds*_____   f. nasal _____*nose*_____
                      glottis

c. dental _teeth_   g. alveolar _alveolar ridge_

d. velar _velum; soft palate_ h. palatal _palate_

2. List the supralaryngeal structures. _tongue, teeth, palate, etc_

3. List the sublaryngeal structures. _trachea, lungs, etc_

4. Name the structure associated with the function/location listed.

   a. Larynx suspended from it _hyoid bone_

   b. Protects larynx in swallowing _epiglottis_

   c. Anterior attachment for vocal folds _thyroid_

   d. Space between vocal folds _glottis_

   e. Responsible for vocal fold abduction _aritenoid cartilage_

   f. Most inferior cartilage, attached to the trachea _____

   g. Muscular tissue shelves _vocal folds_

5. Trace the pathway for a respiratory cycle. List the structures and actions.

6. Define frequency and intensity and name the acoustic products associated with them. _Hz = pitch   db = loudness_

7. From memory, label the structures indicated on this diagram:

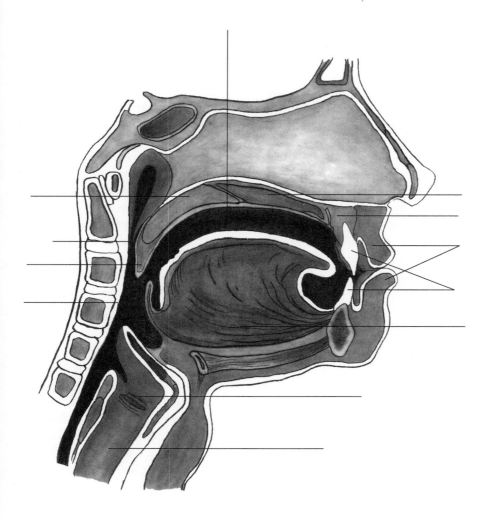

CHAPTER 3

OVERVIEW: VOWELS AND CONSONANTS

ROLE IN SYLLABLE FORMATION
DEGREE OF VOCAL TRACT CONSTRICTION
TRADITIONAL CLASSIFICATION SCHEMES
DISTINCTIVE FEATURE CLASSIFICATION
REVIEW VOCABULARY
EXERCISES

Speech sounds, or phonemes, traditionally have been divided into two categories: consonants and vowels (with diphthongs considered a special kind of vowel). Although this distinction appears relatively straightforward, many phoneticians have disagreed over the actual definitions and identities of the phonemes in each category. They point out that many consonants are nearly indistinguishable from vowels. To be sure, some consonant-vowel categorizations are easy, for example, the /s/ and /o/ in *so*. But many consonants resemble vowels in characteristics such as voicing and oral resonance. A particularly good example of similarities between consonants and vowels can be found with the consonants /w/ (as in *wing*) and /j/ (as in *yes*). These two consonants are actually very similar to the vowels /u/ (as in *boot*) and /i/ (as in *each*) acoustically. They also resemble vowels in their onset of formation; that is, /j/ begins in a position very similar to /i/, and /w/ begins in a position very similar to /u/. (See the section Approximants/Oral Resonant Consonants in Chapter 5 for a full explanation.) Like vowels, /w/ and /j/ are voiced and produced with velopharyngeal closure. Nevertheless, there are several ways that phoneticians typically distinguish vowels from consonants: role in syllable formation, degree of vocal tract constriction, and classification schemes.

ROLE IN SYLLABLE FORMATION

One of the more commonly used and agreed upon ways to distinguish between vowels and consonants is based on their role in syllable formation. With few exceptions, only vowels can form a syllable nucleus. (We will cover the exceptions later, in Chapter 6.) A vowel alone can constitute a syllable, for example, /o/ (*oh*); consonants need not but can be added to it, for example, /go/ (*go*). It is the presence of a vowel, not the consonant, that is necessary to make a syllable. However, if a word contains two vowels, for example, /igo/ (*ego*), then it also consists of two syllables.

DEGREE OF VOCAL TRACT CONSTRICTION

A second, generally accepted way to distinguish between vowels and consonants is based on the degree of constriction, or closure, in the vocal tract. Vowels are produced with a relatively open or unconstricted vocal tract that does not change. Consonants, however, are produced with constriction in the vocal tract. We will illustrate this with an example you should try for yourself. As you produce the sounds that follow, pay close attention to your tongue and jaw position, the tongue movement (or lack of it), and the closeness of your tongue to your palate and alveolar ridge. Now, produce the vowel /ɑ/ (as in *hop*). Next, try to prolong an /s/. What you should notice is that your jaw is much lower and your mouth is more open for vowel production. Also, your tongue tip is very close to your alveolar ridge for the consonant production, but not for the vowel. Now, not all vowels are as "open" as /ɑ/, nor are all consonants as constricted as /s/ (some consonants actually briefly block the airstream). But they do demonstrate the principle that, relatively speaking, the vocal tract is much more open (less constricted) for vowel production than for consonant production.

TRADITIONAL CLASSIFICATION SCHEMES

Within this traditional system, vowels and consonants have separate classification schemes (see Figure 3–1 and Table 3–1). Vowels are classified on the basis of tongue position (front, central, or back) and degree of elevation (high, mid, or low), with some supplemental notation for lip rounding. You will learn to classify consonants in a different way, in terms of their place, manner, and **voicing** characteristics. **Place of articulation** refers to the location of the articulators involved (e.g., alveolar or palatal). **Manner of articulation** is the way in which the airstream is modified (e.g., narrowed [/s/] vs. blocked [/t/]). Finally, consonants are considered **voiced** or voiceless, depending on whether or not the vocal folds are vibrating. These traditional categories will be a primary focus as

POINT OF TONGUE ELEVATION

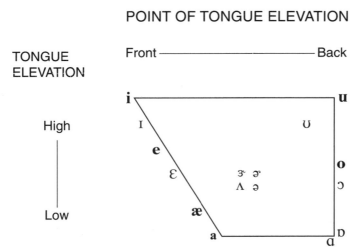

Figure 3–1 *Vowel sounds ordered by tongue elevation and position in the oral cavity. Adapted from the International Phonetic Association (2002).*

TABLE 3–1 CONSONANT SOUNDS OF AMERICAN ENGLISH BY PLACE AND MANNER OF ARTICULATION

Manner of production	Place of Articulation						
	Bilabial	Labio-dental	Lingua-dental	Lingua-alveolar	Lingua-palatal	Lingua-velar	Glottal
Stops	p b			t d		k g	
Fricatives	ʍ	f v	θ	s z	ʃ ʒ	(ʍ)	h
Affricates					tʃ ʤ		
Nasals	m			n		ŋ	
Liquids				l	r		
Glides	w				j	(w)	

( ), secondary articulatory feature

you progress through this book. However, there is another way to classify and distinguish phonemes that we will discuss briefly in the next section of this chapter.

DISTINCTIVE FEATURE CLASSIFICATION

A more recent way to classify phonemes has been through the use of **distinctive features** (see Table 3–2), as described by Noam Chomsky and Morris Halle (1968). Distinctive features are based on both articulatory and acoustic characteristics of phonemes. In contrast, the traditional classifications depend only on the articulatory gestures. Distinctive features actually share many characteristics with the traditional consonant and vowel classification systems that we discussed previously.

In distinctive feature classification systems, each phoneme is viewed as a "bundle" of features. The features themselves are binary, and each phoneme will have (indicated by +) or not have (indicated by −) a particular feature. For example, look for the feature nasal in Table 3–2. As you go across that row, you will find only three phonemes that possess that characteristic, that is, that are classified as + nasal: /m/ /n/ /ŋ/. Thus, the feature nasal corresponds to the traditional manner of articulation, also referred to as nasal. Using distinctive features, a number of consonants are + consonantal (see Table 3–2). The vowels and the two consonants /w/ and /j/ are considered −consonantal, however. Phonemes that are + consonantal have either total closure or extreme narrowing (producing friction) in the oral cavity. The vowels and the consonants /w/ and /j/ are produced with a much more open vocal tract, which makes them −consonantal. (Recall that we noted similarities between the vowels and /w/ and /j/ earlier.)

Distinctive features, then, allow one to classify all phonemes with one system rather than having one method for vowels and another for consonants. Nevertheless, the traditional system introduced first in this chapter is the more frequently used, particularly in the field of applied phonetics. Consequently, we will introduce the phonemes according to traditional consonant and vowel classifications and subclassfications throughout this book.

TABLE 3–2 SELECTED PHONEMES DISTRIBUTED ACCORDING TO 10 DISTINCTIVE FEATURE PROPERTIES OF CHOMSKY AND HALLE (1968)

Phoneme

Feature	b	d	k	f	v	θ	s	z	ʃ	h	tʃ	m	n	ŋ	r	l	w	i	æ	u	a
Sonorant	−	−	−	−	−	−	−	−	−	−	−	+	+	+	+	+	+	+	+	+	+
Consonantal	+	+	+	+	+	+	+	+	+	+	+	+	+	+	+	+	−	−	−	−	−
Vocalic	−	−	−	−	−	−	−	−	−	−	−	−	−	−	+	+	−	+	+	+	+
Coronal	−	+	−	−	−	+	+	+	+	−	+	−	+	−	+	+	−	−	−	−	−
Anterior	+	+	−	+	+	+	+	+	−	−	−	+	+	−	−	+	−	−	−	−	−
Nasal	−	−	−	−	−	−	−	−	−	−	−	+	+	+	−	−	−	−	−	−	−
High	−	−	+	−	−	−	−	−	+	−	+	−	−	+	−	−	+	+	−	+	−
Low	−	−	−	−	−	−	−	−	−	+	−	−	−	−	−	−	−	−	+	−	+
Back	−	−	+	−	−	−	−	−	−	−	−	−	−	+	−	−	−	−	−	+	+
Strident	−	−	−	+	+	−	+	+	+	−	+	−	−	−	−	−	−	−	−	−	−

REVIEW VOCABULARY

distinctive features   acoustic and articulatory characteristics used to distinguish phonemes; features are binary (+ / −).

manner of articulation   refers to the way the airstream is modified for consonant formation.

place of articulation   refers to the place of the airstream modification for consonant formation.

voicing   refers to the presence of vocal fold vibration.

voiced   phoneme produced with vocal fold vibration.

voiceless/unvoiced   phoneme produced without vocal fold vibration.

EXERCISES

1. Using Figure 3–1, list all the back vowels from high to low. _____
_____

2. Using Figure 3–1, list all the front vowels from low to high. _____
_____

3. List all the central vowels. _____
_____

4. Give the place of articulation for the following consonant groups:
   a. /bmp/ _____
   b. /kg/ _____
   c. /ʃtʃʤ/ _____
   d. /stln/ _____

5. Give the manner of articulation for the following consonant groups:
   a. /sfʃθh/ _____
   b. /pdgk/ _____
   c. /wj/ _____
   d. /mn/ _____
   e. /tʃʤ/ _____

6. Using Table 3–2, list the phonemes that are classified as the following:
   a. + coronal _____
   b. − anterior _____
   c. + strident _____
   d. + back _____
   e. + high _____

VOWELS AND DIPHTHONGS

NATURE OF VOWELS

Although both vowels and consonants are phonemes, their formation differs in several ways, as we noted in Chapter 3. American English consonants can differ in place and manner of articulation as well as in voicing. American English vowels, however, are all formed with essentially the same manner of production. They are produced with oral resonance, and they are also all voiced. Vowel identity is primarily a product of shaping of the oral cavity. Oral cavity shape for vowel formation is affected primarily by movements of the tongue, but jaw opening/closing and lip rounding also play a role. American English vowel categorization therefore traditionally has been based on height and placement of tongue elevation with supplemental notation for lip rounding and tenseness. We measure tongue height in tongue-to-palate or tongue-to-velum distance. In articulating vowels from high to low, your jaw movement and tongue position will change vertically because the tongue follows the vertical movement of the mandible. When grouped by place of tongue elevation, the vowels fall into three primary classes: front, back, and central. Consequently, traditional analysis of vowels follows the classification of front, back, or central.

Lip position is noted especially for the rounded vowels /uʊɔ/ and the highly retracted vowels such as /i/. **Tenseness** (and its opposite characteristic, **laxness**) refers to the degree of muscular effort as well as the duration involved in articulating a particular vowel. We will include these characteristics in addition to the primary place and height categories as we discuss each vowel.

Before we introduce the individual vowels and diphthongs, it is important for you to understand the distinction between them. The front, back, and central vowels are **monophthong** vowels; that is, they are produced with one, unchanged (mono-) position. **Diphthongs** involve a transition from one vowel position (**onglide/nucleus**) to another vowel position (**offglide**). There are two vowels that can be monophthongal or diphthongal in mainstream American English: the higher-mid front /e/ (diphthong /eɪ/) and the higher-mid back vowel /o/ (diphthong /ou/). The diphthong forms occur in stressed syllables ([beɪt] or *bait,* [koum] or *comb*). The monophthong form typically is used in syllables with secondary stress, for example, [dɛked] or *de´cade,* [d oneɪ´ʃə n] or *donation.* We will introduce /e/ and /o/ with monophthong vowels but save their transcription for the part of this chapter dealing specifically with diphthongs.

TRADITIONAL ANALYSIS OF VOWELS

The vowel and diphthong phonemes of American English are described individually in the following pages. Front vowels will be introduced first, followed by back vowels, central vowels, and diphthongs. Each vowel will be described in terms of tongue height, placement, lip shape (where applicable), and tenseness/laxness, followed by a step-by-step analysis of production. The appropriate IPA symbol, key words, and examples are supplied for each vowel and diphthong. You will also find additional information about some of the vowels, especially those that are more affected by dialectic variation.

FRONT VOWELS

The front vowels of American English, in order of their tongue height, are /i/, /ɪ/, /e/, /ɛ/, and /æ/. The tongue tip lies just behind and usually touches the inner surface of the mandibular incisors. At the same time, the front or blade of the tongue is raised toward the palate without touching it, and without approximating it closely enough to cause air turbulence or frication (see Figure 4–1). The appropriate tongue-to-palate distance for each vowel can be achieved in several ways: differential elevation of the front tongue in relationship to the (stationary) mandible or holding the front tongue in a high steady position and raising or lowering the

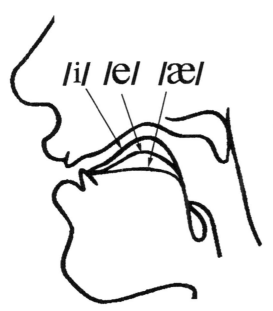

Figure 4–1 Front vowel tongue positions: high to low.

mandible, or some combination of both. You can see this yourself if you try these ways of producing the front vowels. You will need a mirror so that you can watch your lips and jaw. First, hold your mandible in one position by putting a pencil eraser between your front teeth. Now say the front vowels from high to low: /i/ /ɪ/ /e/ /ɛ/ /æ/. Next, begin again with the same tongue and jaw opening for producing /i/ (you can remove the pencil eraser). Try to hold your tongue in a fixed position, and again say these vowels from high to low by dropping your jaw in progressive steps. Did you see your jaw move? You were able to produce the front vowels either way; you simply changed from tongue motion to jaw motion to make it happen. Do not be surprised if you find that one way feels easier or more natural than the other. Either way is appropriate, however. In connected speech, the tongue height for front vowels may be achieved by a combination of tongue and mandible adjustments.

/i/

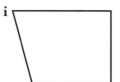

IPA symbol: /i/

Description: high, front, retracted, tense

Key words: eat, seed, be

Common spellings: e, ee, ea, -y

/i/ Production

The velopharyngeal port is closed, and the sides of the back of the tongue are closed against the upper molars. The middle to front portion is raised high, nearly touching the palate and the alveolar ridge. Simultaneously, the tongue tip touches lightly behind the lower front teeth, and voice is given. The upper and lower front teeth are slightly open and the lips tend to be retracted at the corners.

/i/ Words

Initial		Medial		Final	
eat	either	seed	read	be	trustee
eve	Easter	leave	feet	he	free
eel	equal	believe	green	key	tea
east	eager	teach	bead	three	see
each	enough	these	chief	plea	money
even	eagle	lease	sheep	knee	candy

/i/ Sentences

1. The seamstress made sure that all seams were even.
2. She was relieved to find the keys in the Jeep.
3. Dr. Keene is a dean at Elon College.
4. He was very pleased to introduce the board of trustees.
5. Two of the three phonemes in bean and bee are the same.

/i/ Contrasts

/i/–/ɪ/		/i/–/ɛ/	
deep	dip	meat	met
deed	did	bead	bed
beat	bit	neat	net
peak	pick	seat	set
bean	bin	mean	men
peach	pitch	teen	ten

Additional Notes

/i/ has the highest tongue position of the front vowels. It is sometimes modified to /ɪ/, depending on phonetic context and conventions of transcription; for example, the high vowel in *hear* is usually produced as /ɪ/, [h ɪ r].

/ɪ/

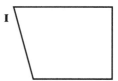

IPA symbol: /ɪ/

Description: (lower) high, front, slightly retracted, lax

Key words: if, bit, mitten

Common spellings: i, y

/ɪ/ Production

The velopharyngeal port is closed, and the sides of the back of the tongue are closed against the upper molars. The middle to front portion is raised toward the palate and alveolar ridge, slightly lower and farther back than for the /i/. Simultaneously, the tongue tip touches lightly behind the lower front teeth, and voice is given. The tongue is less tense than for /i/, and the lips are not as retracted.

/ɪ/ Words

Initial		**Medial**	
in	into	his	pill
it	ignorant	busy	quill
if	interest	limb	sit
id	insect	mitt	tin
ill	idiom	nick	victor

/ɪ/ Sentences

1. The mittens are too little to fit him.
2. The insect is sitting very still.
3. Six inches isn't very big.
4. The crystal shimmered in the light.
5. Is it in this tin?

/ɪ/ Contrasts

/ɪ/	/i/	/ɛ/
bin	bean	Ben
sit	seat	set
gin	gene	Jen
tin	tin	ten
lift	leafed	left
kin	keen	Ken
list	least	lest
chick	cheek	check

Additional Notes

/ɪ/ is one of the most frequently occurring vowels in American English. It is not produced in the final position of words except for unstressed final *y* in some speakers of New England and Southern American English.

/e/

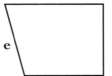

IPA symbol: /e/

Description: (higher-) mid, front, tense

Key words: fatality, vacation, chaotic

Common spelling: a (in syllables not receiving primary stress)

/e/ Production

The velopharyngeal port is closed, and the sides of the back of the tongue are closed against the upper molars. The middle and front portion of the tongue is raised toward the palate and the alveolar ridge, slightly lower and farther back than for the /ɪ/. At the same time, the tongue tip touches lightly behind the lower front teeth. The upper and lower front teeth are open. (If the lips move from this position to an /ɪ/ position, then the diphthong /eɪ/ is produced. See Additional Notes and the section Analysis of Diphthongs for further details and clarification.)

/e/ Words

This symbol is used to transcribe only the vowel of syllables that do not receive primary stress and/or occur at the end of words; its diphthong form, /eɪ/, occurs much more often.

crybaby	fatality
cavalcade	vacation
operate	chaotic
excavate	creativity

/e/ Sentences

See section on /eɪ/ diphthongs in this chapter.

/e/ Contrasts

See section on /eɪ/ diphthongs in this chapter.

Additional Notes

The diphthong form of this vowel occurs much more frequently than the monophthong form. Phoneticians vary in their views and transcription of these forms. As with other vowels, there will be variation between these two forms depending on speech context and dialectic variation. For further details and information, see the section on the /eɪ/ diphthong later in this chapter.

/ɛ/

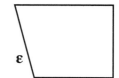

IPA symbol: /ɛ/

Description: (lower-) mid, front, slightly retracted, lax

Key words: end, bet

Common spelling: e

/ɛ/ Production

The velopharyngeal port is closed, and the sides of the back of the tongue are closed against the upper molars. The middle to front portion of the tongue is raised slightly toward the palate and the alveolar ridge, but lower and farther back than for /ɪ/ or /e/. At the same time, the tongue tip touches lightly behind the lower front teeth, and voice is given. The upper and lower front teeth are open slightly wider than for /ɪ/.

/ɛ/ Words

/ɛ/ does not occur in the final position.

	Initial		Medial
edge	extra	men	head
end	elephant	bed	said
egg	else	get	many
elm	engine	them	friend
every	excel	beg	guest
any	effort	neck	bear

/ɛ/ Sentences

1. Many of them said that Ed would be elected.
2. Tell Meg's friend about the ten pets.
3. Don't forget to tell them the directions.
4. You'll have to expend extra effort to excel.
5. Ben likes scrambled eggs for breakfast.

/ɛ/ Contrasts

/ɛ/	/ɪ/	/æ/
send	sinned	sand
bet	bit	bat
lest	list	last
N	in	an
neck	nick	knack
said	Sid	sad
den	din	Dan
met	mitt	mat

Additional Notes

Like /ɪ/, /ɛ/ is one of the most frequently occurring speech sounds in American English speech. It may be pronounced as /ɪ/ in certain dialects, for example, Southern and Appalachian English (see Chapter 8).

/æ/

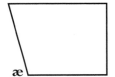

IPA symbol: /æ/

Description: low, front, lax

Key words: at, has

Common spelling: a

/æ/ Production

The velopharyngeal port is closed, and the mouth is open wider than for the other front vowels. The middle to front portion of the tongue is raised lower and farther back than for the other front vowels. The sides of the back of the tongue may move away from the upper molars, and the tongue tip may move slightly behind the lower front teeth.

/æ/ Words

/æ/ does not occur at the end of words in American English.

Initial		Medial	
axe	add	cat	cabin
aunt	Adam	sand	sang
aft	answer	laugh	rather
atom	absolute	that	grant
ask	agony	dance	salmon

/æ/ Sentences

1. The black cat sat in the grass.
2. Dad found some more stamps in the bag.

3. The sand at the beach was damp from the rain.
4. Both Ann and Adam had the right answer to the question.
5. Saturday is the last chance to buy fresh salmon.

/æ/ Contrasts

/æ/	/ɛ/	/ɑ/
add	Ed	odd
had	head	hod
Dan	den	Don
pat	pet	pot
sad	said	sod
panned	penned	pond
gnat	net	knot
banned	bend	bond

Additional Notes

The /æ/ is usually in an accented syllable of a polysyllabic word. It may sound closer to /eɪ/ when it occurs before a nasal consonant (e.g., *kangaroo, rang*). Like other vowels, /æ/ production can vary as a product of context and dialect. In particular, the "New England *a*" (/ɒ/) is a common alternate pronunciation for /æ/ in the northeastern United States (see Chapter 8).

BACK VOWELS

The back vowels of mainstream American English, in order of tongue height, are /u/, /ʊ/, /o/, /ɔ/, and /ɑ/. For back vowels, the back of the tongue is raised toward the velum near its junction with the soft palate (see Figure 4–2). At its high point, the tongue does not touch the velum, nor does it come close enough to cause

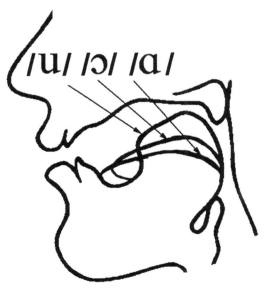

Figure 4–2 Back vowel tongue positions: high to low.

air turbulence or audible friction. The tongue tip rests behind and slightly below the mandibular incisors or lightly touches the lower gum ridge. Like the front vowels, the tongue-to-velum distance needed for each back vowel results from a combination of lingual and mandibular adjustments. With decreasing tongue elevation, the point of back tongue elevation becomes slightly farther forward in the mouth. The higher the tongue, the more rounded the lips. As the highest back vowel, /u/ has the most lip rounding and the smallest lip opening. Conversely, /ɑ/, the low back vowel, is unrounded (but not retracted, like the front vowels). The /ɑ/ has the greatest jaw opening of all the mainstream American English vowel sounds. Look at your mouth in a mirror as you produce the back vowels from high /u/ to low /ɑ/; notice the changes in degree of mouth opening and lip rounding.

/u/

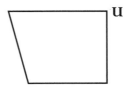

IPA symbol: /u/

Description: high, back, rounded, tense

Key words: ooze, boot, too/to/two

Common spelling: oo

/u/ Production

The velopharyngeal port is closed, and the sides of the back of the tongue are closed against the upper molars. The back of the tongue is raised high and tense, nearly touching the palate. The lips are rounded and may be slightly protruded, producing a small opening. Voice is given. The tongue tip is just behind the lower front teeth, and the upper and lower teeth are slightly open.

/u/ Words

Initial	Medial		Final	
oodles	boot	moon	too	do
ooze	crew	move	who	drew
oolong	doom	rude	Q	blew
oops	fruit	tomb	shoe	through
	group	school	you	flu
	lose	whom	true	canoe

/u/ Sentences

1. Ruth's soup soon grew cool.
2. Lou and Susan went to the pool.
3. Do you want to be in Group One or Group Two?
4. Luke's upper tooth was loose.
5. June is the month that school closes and the pool opens.

/u/ Contrasts

/u/	–	/ʊ/
pool		pull
fool		full
stewed		stood
shooed		should
kook		cook
Luke		look
cooed		could
who'd		hood

Additional Notes

A few words may vary in pronunciation with either /u/ or /ʊ/, depending on the speaker's dialect (e.g., *roof, hoof, root*).

/ʊ/

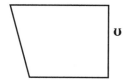

IPA symbol: /ʊ/

Description: (lower) high, back, rounded, lax

Key words: cook, pull, should

Common spellings: oo, u

/ʊ/ Production

The velopharyngeal port is closed, and the sides of the back of the tongue are closed lightly against the upper molars. The back of the tongue is raised high, but lower and with less tension than for /u/. The lips are rounded and may be slightly protruded, producing an opening larger than for /u/. Voice is given. The tongue tip touches behind the lower front teeth, and the upper and lower teeth are slightly open.

/ʊ/ Words

/ʊ/ occurs only in the medial position of words.

Medial

cook	hood	pull
look	woolen	bush
hook	wooden	could
shook	full	should
good	put	would
stood	push	wolf

/ʊ/ Sentences

1. He took the recipe from the cook book.
2. She pushed and pulled the wooden toy.

3. The cook made a jar full of cookies.

4. Put the book here on the good shelf.

5. Could Jim look for the hooks that I put in the garage?

/ʊ/ Contrasts

See /oʊ/ in Analysis of Diphthongs for contrast drills.

Additional Notes

As previously noted, /ʊ/ occurs only in the medial position of words. It can vary with /u/ in production of some words, depending on the speaker's dialect.

/o/

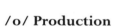

IPA symbol /o/

Description: (higher) mid, front, tense

Key words: donation, location

Most common spelling: o (in syllables not receiving primary stress)

/o/ Production

The velopharyngeal port is closed, and the back and middle portions of the tongue are slightly raised, with elevation slightly lower and more forward than for /ʊ/. The tongue tip touches behind the lower front teeth, and voice is given. The upper and lower front teeth are open. (If the lips and tongue move from this position and briefly assume the position for /ʊ/, then the diphthong /oʊ/ is produced.) The relationship between /o/ and /oʊ/ is similar to that of /e/ and /eɪ/. See Additional Notes and the section Analysis of Diphthongs for further details and clarification.

/o/ Words

This symbol is used to transcribe only the vowel that occurs in syllables that do not receive primary stress and/or occur at the end of words; its diphthong form, /oʊ/, occurs much more often.

innovation	utmost
momentous	cooperate
proliferate	nobility
Cochise	professional

/o/ Sentences

See section on /oʊ/ diphthongs.

/o/ Contrasts

See section on /oʊ/ diphthongs.

Additional Notes

The diphthong form of this vowel occurs much more frequently than the monophthong form. Phoneticians vary in their views and transcription of these forms. As with other vowels, there will be variation between these two forms depending on context and dialectic variations. Further information will be found in the section on the /oʊ/ diphthong later in this chapter.

/ɔ/

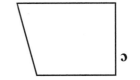

IPA symbol: /ɔ/

Description: (lower) mid, back, rounded, tense

Key words: awful, caught, law

Common spellings: au, aw

/ɔ/ Production

The velopharyngeal port is closed, and the back and middle portions of the tongue are slightly raised, with elevation just below that for /o/. The mouth is open wider than for /o/ production, and the lips are rounded and slightly protruded. Voice is given. The tongue tip touches behind the lower front teeth.

/ɔ/ Words

The /ɔ/ occurrence is very much affected by a speaker's dialect; see Additional Notes for more information.

Initial		Medial		Final	
awful	always	taut	caught	saw	straw
awning	off	applaud	taught	raw	craw
audio	awesome	vault	thought	paw	thaw
auction	often	talk	cloth	caw	gnaw
off	awestruck	walk	wrong	jaw	slaw
auger	almost	yawn	bought	law	raw

/ɔ/ Sentences

1. They all applauded after the talk.
2. I thought that you bought all the cloth you would need.
3. They almost walked the wrong way.
4. He taught a class on law enforcement.
5. They all thought they saw her yawn.

/ɔ/ Contrasts

See next section, /ɑ/, for additional contrasts.

/ɔ/–/oʊ/		/ɔ/–/oʊ/	
bought	boat	fall	foal
taught	tote	caught	coat
paws	pose	jaw	Joe
walk	woke		

Additional Notes

The /ɔ/ is one of the most inconsistently used vowels in American English speech. Compared with /ɑ/, the low back vowel, /ɔ/ differs only by having a slightly higher tongue elevation and lip rounding. /ɔ/ is contrasted consistently from /ɑ/ in some regional American English dialects but is almost always replaced by /ɑ/ in others. The presence or lack of differentiation of /ɔ/ from /ɑ/ across dialects does not appear to have a significant effect on understandability.

/ɑ/

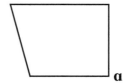

IPA symbol: /ɑ/

Description: low, back, open, lax

Key words: top, cotton, bother

Common spelling: o

/ɑ/ Production

The velopharyngeal port is closed, and the tongue is slightly raised in the back, with the tip touching behind the lower front teeth. The mouth is open wider than for any other vowel as voice is given. The lips are not rounded or protruded but may be described as slightly retracted. /ɑ/ differs primarily from the neutral vowel /ʌ/ in having a wider mouth opening and lower back of tongue elevation.

/ɑ/ Words

The /ɑ/ occurs in final position only in slang words such as *pa* and *ha*. Some of the following words may be produced as /ɔ/ by some speakers.

Initial		**Medial**	
on	obvious	father	Tom
onset	Olive	copper	beyond
honor	ominous	bomb	Bob
odder	oxen	calm	doll
Oz	onyx	Don	psalm
opera	October	Mom	stop

/ɑ/ Sentences

1. Lara and Bob appeared calm.
2. The top was made of cotton, bonded by thread.
3. Olive and palm trees grow in that climate.

4. The tot did not seem to like the new doll.

5. Ron replanted the palm in a new pot.

/ɑ/ Contrasts

/ɑ/	/ɔ/	/oʊ/
cot	caught	coat
not	naught	note
rot	wrought	wrote
hocks	hawks	hoax
mod	Maude	mode

/ɑ/	/ʌ/	/æ/
Bonn	bun	ban
cot	cut	cat
lock	luck	lack
don	done	Dan
mod	mud	mad

Additional Notes

The /ɑ/ is quite variable in American English, often interchanged with /ɔ/ and /æ/. The broad *a* of some Eastern speakers makes words like *aunt* and *bath* be pronounced as [ɒnt] and [bɒθ]. (See the sections Centering Diphthongs in this chapter, Liquid Consonants in Chapter 5, and Chapter 8 for more information and clarification.)

CENTRAL VOWELS

There are four central vowels in American English: /ɝ/, /ɚ/ (stressed and unstressed vowel -*er*) and /ʌ/, /ə/ (stressed and unstressed short ŭ). They are produced with more central tongue elevation; hence the term *central vowels*. The /ʌ/ is the vowel heard in monosyllabic words and stressed syllables such as *mud* and *running,* respectively. The /ə/, occurring in unstressed syllables, is the first vowel in words such as *around* and *unhappy.* The /ɝ/ and /ɚ/ are also referred to as *r*-colored or **rhotacized** vowels. /ɝ/ is the vowel heard in monosyllabic words such as *hurt* and stressed syllables, as in *certain* and *purchase.* The unstressed counterpart, /ɚ/, occurs in words such as *hammer* and *over.* Because of their r-coloring, these vowels may be confused with postvocalic /r/ or /ɚ/ diphthongs, for example, *per* (/pɝ/) versus *pear* (transcribed as /pɛr/). You will find further explanations in the following text and in Chapter 4 in the accompanying workbook.

/ʌ/

IPA symbol: /ʌ/

Description: (lower) mid, central, stressed

Key words: cup, done, rough

Common spelling: u

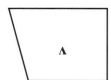

/ʌ/ Production

With the velopharyngeal port closed, the tongue is slightly elevated in the middle to back portion. The upper and lower front teeth are separated about the same distance as for /ɛ/. The tongue tip touches lightly behind the lower front teeth. The airstream is voiced. Because the tongue is in a somewhat relaxed position, /ʌ/ has also been called a "neutral" vowel. This vowel occurs in stressed syllables only.

/ʌ/ Words

Initial		Medial	
upper	upward	cup	flood
upward	utter	tub	blood
under	utmost	hunt	rough
ultimate	oven	some	nothing
other	ugly	done	mother

/ʌ/ Sentences

1. Run and jump in the mud puddle.
2. My uncle got nothing done the other day.
3. Your mother and brother are hunting for something to eat.
4. The usher led the couple into the dining room.
5. The tub was filled with water.
6. They counted one hundred cups in the cupboard.

/ʌ/ Contrasts

/ʌ/–/ɑ/		/ʌ/–/ʊ/		/ʌ/–/ɛ/	
bum	bomb	luck	look	bun	Ben
come	calm	tuck	took	nut	net
gun	gone	stud	stood	but	bet
nut	not	shuck	shook	hull	hell
putt	pot	putt	put	lug	leg
duck	dock	buck	book	mutt	met
cut	cot	cud	could	pun	pen
sum	psalm	crux	crooks	money	many

Additional Notes

This vowel is used for the stressed vowel *uh* in one-syllable words (e.g., *hutch, hum*), in two-syllable words in which the syllable containing /ʌ/ receives primary stress (e.g., *upper, couple, begun*), and in the stressed syllable of polysyllabic words.

/ə/

IPA symbol: /ə/

Description: (lower) mid central vowel, unstressed

Key words: elephant, lemon, sofa

Common spelling: highly variable

/ə/ Production

The velopharyngeal port is closed with tongue placement in the mid-central part of the oral cavity. The tongue is more relaxed than for /ʌ/ production, and duration is shorter than for /ʌ/. The airstream is voiced.

/ə/ Words

Initial		Medial		Final	
about	appeal	alphabet	relative	sofa	vanilla
above	arouse	chocolate	syllable	soda	camera
another	attach	company	emphasis	tuba	gorilla
away	abate	buffalo	accident	quota	arena
awhile	allow	elephant	parasol	zebra	cinema
alive	amaze	parachute	cinnamon	drama	stamina

/ə/ Sentences

1. The woman's stamina was amazing.
2. We saw elephants and zebras at the circus.
3. Hannah liked both vanilla and chocolate soda.
4. Brenda has gone away for awhile.
5. The cinema showed a double feature: a drama and a comedy.

Additional Notes

The /ə/ is also commonly referred to as the schwa vowel. In casual or rapid speech, it is not uncommon for vowels to become /ə/. For example, formal speech would include full pronunciation of all the vowels in *indigo* ([ɪndɪgoʊ]). In rapid, casual speech, the second vowel is most likely to be replaced by /ə/ (e.g., [ɪndəgoʊ]). Because of this tendency, /ə/ is one of the most frequently occurring vowels in English.

/ɝ/

IPA symbol: /ɝ/

Description: mid, central, rounded, tense

Key words: bird, furnace, prefer

Common spelling: er

/ɝ/ Production

The velopharyngeal port is closed, and the sides of the tongue are closed against the upper molars, with the tongue slightly retracted, in a mid-central position. Production is often accompanied by some lip rounding. There are several ways of producing this vowel. The tongue tip may be elevated and curled back toward the alveolar ridge, or the tip may be lowered while the body is bunched near the palate. The airstream is voiced. Duration is longer, and there is more muscular tension than for production of /ɚ/. The /ɝ/ differs from the consonant /r/ in several ways: (1) /ɝ/ has greater duration; (2) /ɝ/ constitutes a syllable; (3) it has tongue movement toward, rather than away from, the consonant /r/ position; and (4) it is never voiceless following voiceless consonants, as /r/ can be.

/ɝ/ Words

Initial		Medial		Final	
earth	earn	pearl	courage	her	stir
early	urchin	sturdy	learn	burr	aver
earl	urn	pertinent	herd	fur	her
earthly	Irving	heard	furnish	purr	sir
irked	earnest	kernel	stern	were	occur
Ernie	urged	work	bird	infer	spur

/ɝ/ Sentences

1. The *early* b*ir*d gets the w*or*m.
2. *Ernie* h*ear*d h*er* coming.
3. The th*ir*d g*ir*l took the f*ir*st t*ur*n.
4. *Lear*ning doesn't occ*ur* without w*or*k.
5. H*er* b*ir*d wakes h*er* *ear*ly every m*or*ning.

/ɝ/ Contrasts

/ɝ/–/ʊ/		/ɝ/–/ʌ/		/ɝ/ or /ɚ/–/r/	
shirk	shook	hurt	hut	terrain	train
stirred	stood	lurk	luck	beret	bray
curd	could	shirk	shuck	duress	dress
lurk	look	shirt	shut	curried	creed
word	wood	pert	putt	per	pear
furl	full	burn	bun	her	hear
gird	good	curt	cut	scurry	scary
Turk	took	burrs	buzz	stir	stair
				worm	warm
				bird	board

Additional Notes

As you may have noticed from the last Discrimination drill, the /ɝ/ may be confused with **rhotic** (r-colored) diphthongs or when consonant /r/ follows a vowel, as in *card* and *bear*. We will discuss these differences further in Analysis of Diphthongs (following pages) and in the Approximants/Oral Resonant Consonants section of Chapter 5. We will save more intense drill on /ɝ/–/ɚ/ as opposed to consonant /r/ discrimination skills until those sections.

/ɚ/

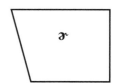

IPA symbol: /ɚ/

Description: mid, central, lax

Key words: brother, Saturday

Common spelling: er (unstressed syllables)

/ɚ/ Production

The velopharyngeal port is closed, and the tongue position is similar to that for /ɝ/. However, /ɚ/ is produced with less muscular tension and is shorter in duration than /ɝ/. The airstream is voiced. This vowel occurs only in unstressed or lightly stressed syllables. Lip rounding occurs often but varies.

/ɚ/ Words

urbane	mother	labor	pewter
martyr	terrain	hammer	gingerbread
understand	improper	gathered	anger
researcher	perchance	emperor	intern

/ɚ/ Sentences

1. My moth*er* and sist*er* are both coming ov*er*.
2. It's a matt*er* of und*er*standing the lab*or* involved.
3. The butt*er* is und*er* the top shelf in the refrig*er*ator.
4. She measu*er*d the sug*ar* for the ging*er*bread.
5. The play*er* hit the ball to cent*er* field.

Additional Notes

The /ɚ/ symbol is similar in appearance to the /ə/. It is sometimes referred to as "schwar." It may be affected by dialectic variation, particularly in New England and the South.

ANALYSIS OF DIPHTHONGS

Like vowels, diphthongs serve as the nucleus of syllables. They are considered single phonemes, each composed of a sequence of vowel positions. One of the positions is the dominant nucleus or onglide, which has greater duration. The nucleus is fol-

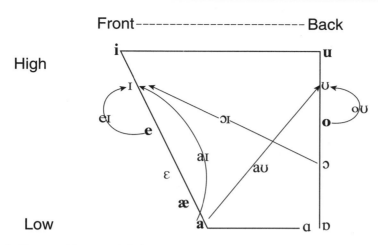

Figure 4–3 *Movements for rising diphthongs.*

lowed by the offglide portion, which has reduced duration and stress relative to the nucleus. Both positions are taken in a single syllable. The traditional, or rising, diphthongs of English are /eɪ/, /oʊ/, /aɪ/, /ɔɪ/, and /aʊ/. Another set of diphthongs, the centering diphthongs, have /ɚ/ as their offglide. Some phoneticians transcribe postvocalic *r*s as centering diphthongs, but more frequently they use consonant /r/, for example, [kɑr] as opposed to [kɑɚ] to transcribe *car*. We discuss both types of diphthongs in this chapter and in the workbook. Ultimately, however, we will use the more common /r/ for *r*, which follows the vowel in our transcription. This will be more understandable when you learn about the liquid consonants /r/ and /l/ in Chapter 5.

Because diphthongs are characterized by movement, they need to be depicted by tongue movement, as in Figures 4–3 and 4–4. These figures use the now familiar vowel diagram to indicate direction of movement from nucleus to offglide position. For traditional diphthongs, movement is from a lower tongue elevation to a higher elevation. For /ɚ/ diphthongs, movement is toward the central vowel position.

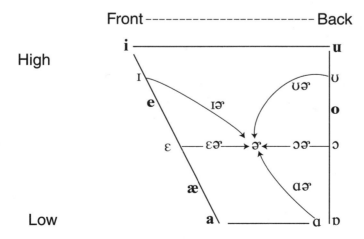

Figure 4–4 *Movements for centering diphthongs.*

RISING DIPHTHONGS

IPA symbols: /eɪ/ /ou/ /aɪ/ /au/ /ɔɪ/

Description: front, rising diphthongs (3)

back, rising diphthongs (2)

Key words: /eɪ/ hay, safer

/ou/ old, gopher

/aɪ/ my, higher

/au/ out, powder

/ɔɪ/ oil, oyster

/eɪ/

IPA symbol: /eɪ/

Description: front, rising diphthong

Key words: able, made, may

Common spelling: a-e

/eɪ/ Production

With the velopharyngeal port closed and the sides of the back of the tongue closed against the upper molars, the middle and front portions of the tongue are raised toward the palate and the alveolar ridge, slightly lower and farther back than for /ɪ/; then the tongue briefly rises toward the /ɪ/ height. The airstream is voiced throughout production. The tongue tip touches lightly behind the lower front teeth. The upper and lower front teeth are open and may move from the /e/ to the /ɪ/ opening. The [e] portion is the longer nucleus, and the [ɪ] portion is the shorter offglide. For many speakers, the glide portion may have a tongue-mouth position close to /i/ but of short duration.

/eɪ/ Words

Initial		Medial		Final	
age	apex	bake	label	may	neigh
ache	eight	came	baby	bay	weigh
aim	alien	date	making	say	decay
aid	aviary	face	placed	spray	away
able	apron	steak	taper	they	matinee
ape	acre	gain	relation	prey	ballet

/eɪ/ Sentences

1. Our neighbor had a baby last Saturday.
2. James and Kate came today.
3. The agent placed the tapes on the tray.

4. They are going away for vacation.

5. They went to the matinee later in the day.

/eɪ/ Contrasts

/eɪ/–/ɛ/		/eɪ/–/ɪ/	
mate	met	mate	mitt
date	debt	late	lit
bait	bet	tame	Tim
rake	wreck	wait	wit
main	men	bait	bit
gate	get	chain	chin
laid	led	fate	fit
fade	fed	hate	hit

Additional Notes

In words like *air* and *care* (vowel followed by postvocalic /r/), the vowel may be heard and transcribed as /eɪ/, /e/, or /ɛ/. The /ɛ/ is the most common variant, particularly if you transcribe with centering diphthongs (e.g., [ɛɚ], [kɛɚ]). In American English, the /eɪ/ usually occurs with a primary accent. It can also occur with a secondary accent if it is in a final open syllable (e.g., *Monday, Saturday*). Use of /e/ tends to be restricted to unaccented syllables that occur next to the accented syllable, for example, the following:

/eɪ/	/e/
na´tive	nati´vity
fa´tal	fata´lity
va´cate	vaca´tion
cha´os	chao´tic

/oʊ/

IPA symbol: /oʊ/

Description: back, rising diphthong

Key words: own, boat, no

Common spelling: -o-e, -oa

/oʊ/ Production

With the velopharyngeal port closed, the middle and back portions of the tongue are raised toward the palate, slightly lower than for /ʊ/. The lips are rounded and may be slightly protruded, with the opening slightly larger than for /ʊ/. The airstream is voiced. The tongue rises briefly to the /ʊ/ height, and the rounded lip opening decreases in size. The tip of the tongue touches lightly behind the lower front teeth. The [o] portion is the longer nucleus, and the [ʊ] is the shorter offglide.

/oʊ/ Words

Initial		Medial		Final	
oak	ocean	boat	toes	go	toe
oats	over	pole	thrown	no	hoe
only	oaf	code	both	so	woe
opal	odor	showed	rose	row	sew
own	omen	broke	hope	low	dough
open	oval	road	smoke	bow	though

/oʊ/ Sentences

1. The crow flew slowly over the road.
2. The boat goes over the ocean.
3. Joe showed the note to Rose.
4. Joan sewed the bow on the coat.
5. Zoe showed us the road that led to the ocean.

/oʊ/ Contrasts

/oʊ/–/ʊ/		/oʊ/–/ɔ/	
pole	pull	phone	fawn
bowl	bull	boat	bought
code	could	coat	caught
showed	should	pose	pause
stowed	stood	tote	taught
goad	good	bowl	bawl
broke	brook	coal	call
coke	cook	foal	fall

Additional Notes

When *o, oa-, o-e,* or other spellings associated with /oʊ/ are followed by post-vocalic /r/, the vowel is more often transcribed as /o/ or /ɔ/, for example, *for* as [for] or [fɔr].

In mainstream English, the /oʊ/ occurs in syllables with a primary accent (e.g., *only, emotion*). /oʊ/ is also used for open, final, unaccented syllables (e.g., wind*ow,* yell*ow.* As noted previously in the section on /o/, the /oʊ/ diphthong occurs much more often than the monophthong /o/. Most often, an unaccented vowel is transcribed as the monophthong /o/ when the sound is in the syllable next to the accented syllables, for example, in the following:

/oʊ/	/o/
ro´tate	rota´tion
lo´cate	loca´tion
do´nate	dona´tion
pro´rate	prora´tion

/aɪ/

IPA symbol: /aɪ/

Description: Back, rising diphthong

Key words: ice, mine, high

Common spellings: i, y, ie, igh

/aɪ/ Production

The velopharyngeal port is closed and the mouth is open as for /æ/, with the middle and front portions of the tongue raised more than for /ʌ/ but less than for /æ/. The tongue rises briefly in front toward the /i/ height, and the mouth opening is slightly decreased. The tip of the tongue touches lightly behind the lower front teeth, and the airstream is voiced throughout production. The [a] portion is the longer nucleus, and the [ɪ] portion is the shorter offglide. For some speakers, the nucleus may be closer to the /ɑ/ position and the offglide close to /i/ but of short duration.

/aɪ/ Words

Initial		Medial		Final	
ice	item	find	light	by	die
ivy	idea	child	psyche	my	lie
idle	icicle	wild	shine	guy	sigh
iris	eyes	kind	fright	deny	bye
aisle	eyed	pine	type	thigh	buy
ivory	island	hide	height	sky	rye

/aɪ/ Sentences

1. Mike tried to fly the kite.
2. My friend Iris likes ice cream.
3. That child's bike is the right size.
4. I'd like to buy five items.
5. Why not take a hike on the island?

/aɪ/ Contrasts

/aɪ/–/ɑ/		/aɪ/–/ɪ/		/aɪ/–/aʊ/	
type	top	ride	rid	dine	down
ride	rod	fine	fin	mice	mouse
pipe	pop	like	lick	nine	noun
like	lock	type	tip	lied	loud
light	lot	sign	sin	by	bow
fire	far	hide	hid	high	how
side	sod	light	lit	file	fowl
hide	hod	bite	bit	spite	spout

/aʊ/

IPA symbol: /aʊ/

Description: back rising diphthong

Key words: out, loud, now

Common spellings: ou, ow

/aʊ/ Production

The velopharyngeal port is closed, and the mouth is opened as for /æ/. The middle and front portions of the tongue are raised more than for /ʌ/ but less than for /æ/. The tongue briefly rises in the back toward the /ʊ/ height, the mouth opening is slightly decreased, and the lips are round as for /ʊ/. The tip of the tongue touches lightly behind the lower front teeth and may move back slightly for the [ʊ] portion. The airstream is voiced throughout production. The [a] portion is the longer nucleus, and the [ʊ] portion is the shorter glide. For some speakers, the nucleus may be closer to the /ɑ/ position and the offglide close to /u/ but of short duration.

/aʊ/ Words

Initial		Medial		Final	
out	outlaw	count	town	now	vow
ouch	outline	found	foul	cow	endow
ounce	outfit	mouse	gown	sow	allow
oust	output	doubt	dowel	prow	somehow
ours	outlet	noun	towel	how	eyebrow
owl	hour	about	brown	bough	thou

/aʊ/ Sentences

1. Count on us for about an hour.
2. I doubt that they found the owl.
3. The crowd downtown was loud.
4. The loud shout meant the player was out.
5. The mouth is rounded for the /ʊ/ portion of the /aʊ/ sound.

/aʊ/ Contrasts

/aʊ/–/ɑ/		/aʊ/–/ʌ/		/aʊ/–/aɪ/	
shout	shot	town	ton	down	dine
spout	spot	down	done	mouse	mice
down	don	gown	gun	noun	nine
cowed	cod	bout	butt	loud	lied
scout	Scott	found	fund	bow	by
gout	got	cowl	cull	how	high
pout	pot	noun	nun	fowl	file

/ɔɪ/

IPA symbol: /ɔɪ/

Description: back, rising diphthong

Key words: oil, coin, boy

Common spellings: oi, oy

/ɔɪ/ Production

The velopharyngeal port is closed, and the back and middle portions of the tongue are slightly raised with elevation as for /ɔ/, while the mouth is open for /ɔ/ with the lips rounded and slightly protruded. The lip rounding then relaxes, and the tongue briefly rises toward the /ɪ/ height. The lower jaw may move upward from the opening of /ɔ/ to the smaller opening of /ɪ/. The [ɔ] is the longer nucleus, and the [ɪ] portion is the shorter offglide. The airstream is voiced throughout production. For many speakers, the glide portion may have a tongue-mouth position close to /i/ but for short duration.

/ɔɪ/ Words

Initial	Medial		Final	
oil	foil	boycott	boy	toy
oiler	coin	royal	soy	deploy
ointment	voice	mastoid	cloy	coy
oyster	join	appoint	joy	enjoy
	soil	goiter	Roy	destroy
	loin	thyroid	poi	Troy

/ɔɪ/ Sentences

1. Roy's voice was noisy and joyous.
2. Troy recommended a boycott of the oil company.
3. The boys would like Roy to play with them and their toys.
4. You will need vegetable oil and soy sauce for the recipe.
5. Poise, joys, and noise are all rhyming words containing the /ɔɪ/ diphthong.

/ɔɪ/ Contrasts

/ɔɪ/–/aɪ/		/ɔɪ/–/ɔ/		/ɔɪ/–/ɝ/	
toil	tile	coil	call	oil	earl
poise	pies	foil	fall	loin	learn
toys	ties	toil	tall	voice	verse
loin	line	boil	ball	boil	burl
foil	file	joy	jaw	poise	purrs
boy	buy	cloy	claw	boys	burrs
voice	vice	noise	gnaws	royal	rural
oil	aisle	soy	saw	coil	curl

Additional Notes

Some dialects may substitute /ɔɪ/ and /ɝ/ in different words; for example, [gɔɪl] for *girl* but [ɝl] for *oil*.

CENTERING DIPHTHONGS /ɪɚ/, /ɛɚ/, /ʊɚ/, /ɔɚ/, AND /ɑɚ/

Description: front, centering diphthongs (2)

back, centering diphthongs (3)

Key words: /ɪɚ/ *ear,* h*ear*e

/ɛɚ/ *air,* c*are*

/ʊɚ/ *sure,* p*ure*

/ɔɚ/ *soar,* p*ore*

/ɑɚ/ *car,* j*ar*

Additional Notes

Because we will be transcribing postvocalic /r/ in consonant form, we will defer listening and transcription of these words until the workbook.

REVIEW VOCABULARY

back vowels   monophthong vowels that involve elevation of the back of the tongue in the oral cavity.

central vowels   monophthong vowels involving elevation or placement of the middle of the tongue in the oral cavity.

diphthong   a single phoneme with a sequence of two different vowel positions, consisting of a dominant nucleus vowel with greater duration and an offglide vowel with reduced duration and stress.

front vowels   monophthong vowels involving raising of the front of the tongue in the oral cavity.

laxness   see Lax vowels.

lax vowels   vowels produced with shorter duration and less tension of the oral musculature.

monophthong   vowel produced with the vocal tract in a fixed position; also known as a "pure" vowel.

nucleus   with reference to diphthongs, the first, dominant articulatory gesture.

onglide   with reference to diphthongs, see Nucleus.

offglide   with reference to diphthongs, the vowel component with reduced duration and stress, following the diphthong nucleus.

rhotacized   refers to positioning or influence of /r/.

round vowels   vowels with resonance influenced by rounding and slight protrusion of the lips (include /u/, /ʊ/, /o/, /ɔ/, and /ɝ/).

tenseness   see Tense vowels.

tense vowels   vowels produced with relatively greater duration and tension in the oral musculature.

EXERCISES

1. Place the following vowels in order of tongue elevation (high to low):
   /ɛ/   /e/   /i/   /æ/   /ɪ/

2. Place the following back vowels in order of tongue elevation (high to low):
   /o/   /ʊ/   /u/   /ɑ/   /ɔ/

3. List the high vowels:

4. List the mid vowels:

5. List the low vowels:

6. What characteristic do the vowels /o/, /ɔ/, /u/, /ɝ/, and /ʊ/ share?

7. From memory, fill in the vowels in this figure, and label the two dimensions:

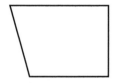

8. Pronounce and transliterate into orthographic alphabet symbols the following vowels:
   /aɪ/   /i/   /oʊ/   /eɪ/

CHAPTER 5

CONSONANTS

ANALYSIS OF CONSONANTS
REVIEW VOCABULARY
EXERCISES

ANALYSIS OF CONSONANTS

As we noted in Chapter 3, **consonants** traditionally have been classified according to three characteristics: place of articulation, manner of articulation, and voicing. Place of articulation refers to the location (e.g., labial, alveolar) of airstream modification or to those parts of the speech mechanism used most prominently in consonant production. You learned the terms to describe place of articulation in Chapter 2. For example, /p/ and /b/ share a *bilabial* place of articulation, whereas /h/ has a *glottal* place of articulation. **Manner of articulation** refers to the way the airstream is modified. You will learn the consonants according to their manner of articulation: **stop, fricative, affricate, nasal,** and **approximant/oral resonant** (**liquids** and **glides**). The third classification category, voicing, refers to vocal fold vibration, as you also learned in Chapter 2. Consonants such as /b/ and /z/, which involve phonation, are voiced, and consonants such as /p/ and /s/, made without phonation, are voiceless.

It is also important to understand the terminology that refers to the role of consonants in relation to vowels. We can refer to consonants as **singletons** (one consonant with no consonants adjacent to it) or **sequences** (two or more consonants in succession in the same syllable or word). We can also refer to consonant singletons or sequences as **prevocalic, intervocalic,** or **postvocalic.** Prevocalic refers to consonant(s) occurring before a vowel, at the beginning of a word, and postvocalic is the term applied to consonant(s) that occur after a vowel, at the end of a word. If a consonant is intervocalic, then it occurs between two vowels in a multisyllabic word. Thus, /p/ is a prevocalic consonant singleton in the word [paɪ] (*pie*), and /sp/ is a prevocalic consonant sequence in the word [spaɪ] (*spy*). The word [p aɪp] (*pipe*) ends with a postvocalic /p/, and the word [p aɪ ps] (*pipes*) ends with a postvocalic consonant sequence. In the word [baɪsɪkəl] (*bicycle*), /s/ is an intervocalic consonant singleton. Corrrespondingly, the /sk/ is an intervocalic consonant sequence in the word [bæskɪt] (*basket*). Older, more traditional terms used to refer to word position are initial, medial, and final.

There are two kinds of consonant sequences: **blends** and **abutting** consonants. Blends consist of two or more adjacent consonants occurring within the same syllable, for example, /bl/ in [blu] (*blue*). Abutting consonants consist of two or more adjacent consonants that cross a syllable boundary, for example, /tp/ in [pɑtpaɪ] (*potpie*). Both blends and abutting consonants are examples of consonant sequences, but they are just two different kinds of sequences. (For more examples of these terms, see Table 5–1.)

The consonant phonemes of American English speech are described individually in this chapter. Their symbols, as used in the International Phonetic Alphabet, key words, and most common spellings, are listed for each symbol. Each consonant production is described in simple place and manner terms and also step by step. These descriptions are followed by examples of words (organized by position), sentences, and contrast discrimination exercises for each consonant. Notes are also added about some phonemes with regard to frequency of occurrence and age of acquisition.

Although these production descriptions may sound absolute or cut-and-dried, this is not really the case, particularly in connected speech. Each description is more a generalization of how most people produce speech sounds. We all make accommodations for our unique anatomy and for our skill in moving the speech mechanism rapidly about. You did not learn speech through careful instruction, carefully watching and copying someone else's tongue or lip movements. Instead, you learned speech by listening and, by trial and error, moving your speech mechanism until you produced a sound that was similar to those of more mature speakers. There is more than one possible way to produce the same sound, and there will be individual differences in the particular way people habitually produce speech. Nevertheless, there are enough common characteristics for us to devise "typical" descriptions. Such descriptions serve as excellent reference points for teaching someone who has not acquired a particular consonant or consonants.

TABLE 5–1 EXAMPLES OF CONSONANT POSITION IN WORDS

Word	Consonant(s)	Singleton/Sequence	Position
Ed [ɛd]	/d/	Singleton	Postvocalic
said [sɛd]	/s/	Singleton	Prevocalic
	/d/	Singleton	Postvocalic
sled [slɛd]	/sl/	Sequence: blend	Prevocalic
sleds [slɛdz]	/dz/	Sequence: blend	Postvocalic
sledding [slɛdɪŋ]	/sl/	Sequence: blend	Prevocalic
	/d/	Singleton	Intervocalic
	/ŋ/	Singleton	Postvocalic
tooth [tuθ]	/t/	Singleton	Prevocalic
	/θ/	Singleton	Postvocalic
toothbrush	/t/	Singleton	Prevocalic
	/θbr/	Sequence: abutting	Intervocalic
	/ʃ/	Singleton	Postvocalic

STOP CONSONANTS

There are six stop consonants in American English: /p/, /t/, /k/, /b/, /d/, and /g/. All are produced with the velopharyngeal port closed. This manner of articulation requires that the voiced or voiceless airstream be interrupted by closure within the oral cavity. The airstream interruption has two possible phases. The stop (or necessary) phase requires rapid closure within the oral cavity. The second, more variable, phase is the **aspiration** (**plosive**) phase, in which the impounded or blocked airstream is released. These two phases have led some phoneticians to refer to this manner of articulation as stop-plosives. Some allophones of stops are made with or without aspiration. Try saying the word *hop* in these two ways: first, release the air (puff of air, stop + aspiration phase) as you produce the /p/ in the word. Next, say *hop,* but keep your lips closed (no air release, stop phase only). Both productions sound like the intended word, but the aspiration phase was not required for meaning. Stops may or may not be released with aspiration in connected speech. We will discuss the different conditions for aspiration in Chapter 6. Each stop will be introduced individually, linked to cognate and place of articulation.

/p/

IPA symbol: /p/

Cognate: /b/

Description: voiceless bilabial stop

Key words: pie, happy, top

Common spellings: p, pp

/p/ Production

The /p/ is made with the velopharyngeal port closed and without voicing. For the necessary stop phase, the lips close, and the breath is held and compressed in the oral cavity. Lip closure for /p/ is made with more tension and greater duration than for /b/. In the variable aspiration or plosive phase, the compressed air is released suddenly as an audible explosion of air between the lips. In connected speech, the /p/ may or may not be released with aspiration.

/p/ Words

Initial		Medial		Final		Sequences	
pack	pool	upon	paper	up	shop	pry	camp
pie	pun	apple	rapid	cap	cape	spring	kept
peas	peak	upper	repair	chop	deep	split	clasp
pill	pot	happy	stopping	ape	mope	pleat	grasps
pine	paint	stupid	oppose	reap	hoop	speak	hopped

/p/ Sentences

1. *Paula* was *proud* of the *paper* she had com*p*leted.
2. They were ha*pp*y to find the *pool* in *p*lace.

3. They are chopping up the pine tree.
4. Paul's favorite dessert is apple pie topped with ice cream.
5. You can put your completed project on top of the pile.
6. Pete used a sponge to mop up the damp part.

/p/ Contrasts

/p/–/b/		/p/–/t/		/p/–/k/	
pack	back	pie	tie	pear	care
pill	Bill	pan	tan	pan	can
peas	bees	pin	tin	peep	keep
rope	robe	pop	pot	lap	lack
tap	tab	rap	rat	seep	seek

Additional Notes

The /p/ is developed early by children and is seldom misarticulated. It occurs less frequently than all the other stops except for /g/ in mainstream American English.

/b/

IPA symbol: /b/

Cognate: /p/

Description: voiced bilabial stop

Key words: be, oboe, cab

Common spellings: b, bb

/b/ Production

The /b/ is made with the velopharyngeal port closed and with voicing. In the necessary stop or closure phase, the lips close as voicing begins or continues, and air is held briefly in the oral cavity. Closure for /b/ is less tense and of shorter duration than for /p/. If the optional release phase then follows, the lips are opened as voicing continues.

/b/ Words

Initial		Medial		Final		Sequences	
be	boot	baby	maybe	tub	orb	blue	rubs
by	bad	robot	nobody	crab	curb	brew	rubbed
bed	boy	about	labor	globe	herb	blaze	number
book	boom	ribbon	hammer	cube	knob	bland	rainbow
bait	bead	pebble	October	bib	lab	bread	tumbler

/b/ Sentences

1. Robins, bluebirds, and blackbirds are all songbirds.
2. Maybe somebody will buy Bill's boat.
3. Bring Ben that big blue book by the chalkboard.
4. The baby blanket had ribbons on the bottom.
5. The brown ball bounced against the floorboards.
6. Bob found a rabbit in the cabbage patch.

/b/ Contrasts

/b/-/p/		/b/-/v/		/b/-/m/		/b/-/d/	
bend	penned	berry	very	bee	me	bore	door
ban	pan	best	vest	best	messed	Ben	den
beat	Pete	boat	vote	by	my	bid	did
tab	tap	gibbon	given	hub	hum	cab	cad
robe	rope	bow	vow	lab	lamb	lab	lad

Additional Notes

The /b/ is mastered early by children and seldom misarticulated. It occurs more frequently in American English than its cognate, /p/. Speakers of English as a second language may show some alterations of /b/. (See Chapter 8, Multicultural Variations: Dialects for more information.)

/t/

IPA symbol: /t/

Cognate: /p̶/ /d/

Description: voiceless (lingua-)alveolar stop

Key words: tie, later, sit

Common spellings: t, tt, -ed

/t/ Production

The /t/ is made with the velopharyngeal port closed and without voice. In the first, (necessary) stop phase, the tip of the tongue closes against the alveolar ridge, with the sides of the tongue against the molars. The breath is held and compressed in the oral cavity at this point. Closure is more tense and of greater duration than for the cognate /d/. In the (optional) aspiration phase, the compressed air behind the tongue is released suddenly as an audible explosion between the alveolar ridge and the tip of the tongue through slightly open teeth and lips.

/t/ Words

Initial		Medial		Final		Sequences	
too	tie	otter	potato	at	eat	trust	gifts
take	tone	pretty	city	cut	wait	treat	waked

Initial		Medial		Final		Sequences	
tube	teak	letter	shouted	gate	goat	twin	stretch
toe	time	rotate	batted	seat	shut	twill	guests
team	tip	meter	gator	plate	pleat	train	paints

/t/ Sentences

1. Tom walked two miles to get the cat.
2. Yesterday Theresa bought a beautiful basket.
3. The twins' names are Ted and Thomas.
4. It took twelve innings for our team to beat them.
5. Did you see what Tanya bought at the store?
6. It's too late to take the two o'clock train.

/t/ Contrasts

/t/–/d/		/t/–/θ/		Singleton-Sequence	
tie	dye	tin	thin	lass	last
ton	done	tick	thick	pass	past
metal	medal	tinker	thinker	slip	slipped
mat	mad	bat	bath	guess	guest
coat	code	boat	both	wash	washed

Additional Notes

/t/ is one of the most frequently occurring sounds in American English. It is mastered early by children in the prevocalic and postvocalic positions. Intervocalic /t/, especially in unstressed syllables, is sometimes produced as a brief, voiced "flap" (/ɾ/) of the tongue, rather than a voiceless stop (e.g., *better, butter, pity, waiting, beautiful*). See Chapter 6 for further information on this topic.

/d/

IPA symbol: /d/

Cognate: /t/

Description: voiced (lingua-)alveolar stop

Key words: day, muddy, fad

Common spellings: d, dd, ed

/d/ Production

/d/ is made with the velopharyngeal port closed and with vocal fold vibration. In the necessary stop phase, the tip of the tongue closes against the alveolar ridge with the sides of the tongue against the molars. Air is held briefly in the oral cavity at this closure. Closure is usually tense and of shorter duration than for /t/. In the optional release phase, the closure of the tongue tip against the alveolar ridge is released while voicing continues.

/d/ Words

Initial		Medial		Final		Sequences	
do	date	somebody	model	bad	owed	dwell	hand
day	dyne	ladder	jaded	did	sued	drain	cards
dog	dine	lady	madder	read	made	drop	razed
dish	deep	lowdown	reader	bird	bead	dwarf	posed
down	deal	nobody	adore	load	amid	dry	bond

/d/ Sentences

1. I wouldn't spend a dime on that dish.
2. Drew handed Dana his new address.
3. They had to herd the reindeer down to the meadow.
4. Mandy has a bad cold.
5. The lady donated a thousand dollars to the fund drive.
6. Fred did all he could to aid the dog.

/d/ Contrasts

/d/–/t/		/d/–/ð/		/d/–/n/	
dying	tying	dine	thine	done	nun
dean	teen	den	then	do	new
medal	metal	fodder	father	madder	manner
riding	writing	seed	seethe	raid	rain
hide	height	breed	breathe	seed	seen

Additional Notes

Like /p/ and /b/, /d/ is mastered fairly early by children. It is misarticulated more often than /p/ and /b/, however. Like /t/, it is one of the most frequently occurring consonants in American English.

/k/

IPA symbol: /k/

Cognate: /g/

Description: voiceless (lingua) velar stop

Key words: key, become, back

Common spellings: k, c, ck

/k/ Production

The velopharyngeal port is closed, and there is no vocal fold vibration throughout /k/ production. In the necessary stop phase, the back of the tongue closes against the front of the velum or back portion of the palate, and the breath is held and compressed in the oral cavity and the oropharynx. If the optional aspiration phase follows, the compressed air is released suddenly between the tongue and the roof of the mouth.

/k/ Words

Initial		Medial		Final		Sequences	
key	come	jacket	stocking	hook	oak	cry	silk
cat	cold	acre	okay	rock	stick	clown	asks
could	count	bucket	bacon	wake	tick	picture	biscuit
coal	caught	become	backache	cake	duck	crow	looked
kite	camp	baker	beacon	peek	rake	creed	thinks

/k/ Sentences

1. *K*en's boo*k* was in his ja*ck*et po*ck*et.
2. It's o*k*ay to as*k* about the pi*c*ture of the *c*at.
3. We had *c*o*c*oa and graham *c*ra*ck*ers for a sna*ck*.
4. Did *K*athy ba*k*e *c*ake or *c*ookies for the pi*c*ni*c*?
5. The s*c*outs helped to *c*lean up the par*k* for *c*amping.
6. *K*ay's sto*ck* mar*k*et in*c*ome is rising.

/k/ Contrasts

/k/–/g/		/k/–/t/		/k/–/p/	
cap	gap	cone	tone	care	pear
coat	goat	came	tame	cool	pool
cab	gab	hack	hat	cat	pat
bicker	bigger	ache	ate	coke	cope
rack	rag	scare	stare	seek	seep

Additional Notes

/k/ is acquired fairly early by children, but later than /p/ and /b/. It is not usually misarticulated unless a child has a hearing loss or a phonological problem. When it is misarticulated, it is most often replaced by /t/. /k/ is one of the most frequently occurring American English consonants, but not as frequent as /t/.

/g/

IPA symbol: /g/

Cognate: /k/

Description: voiced (lingua) velar stop

Key words: go, foggy, log

Common spellings: g, gg

/g/ Production

The /g/ is made with the velopharyngeal port closed and with vocal fold vibration. In the necessary stop phase, the back of the tongue closes against the front of the velum or the back portion of the palate, and air is held briefly in the back of the oral cavity and the oropharynx. Closure is less tense and of shorter duration than for /k/. In the variable release phase, the closure of the back of the tongue against the velum or palate is released as voicing continues.

/g/ Words

Initial		Medial		Final		Sequences	
go	guest	again	buggy	egg	vague	glass	finger
gate	give	begin	bigger	dog	rogue	green	giggling
gun	geese	ago	logger	tug	intrigue	grow	single
good	ghost	ego	bagger	bag	tag	Gwen	sags
gap	gasp	beggar	sagging	dig	big	gleam	bugged

/g/ Sentences

1. The big gray goose is gone.
2. Guy and Gary argued again.
3. Gwen found the guys grooming the dog.
4. Greg forgot the grapes by the gate.
5. He put his garden gloves together by the gate.
6. Clean off that grungy dog and don't let him dig again.

/g/ Contrasts

/g/–/k/		/g/–/d/		/g/–/ŋ/	
gain	cane	guy	dye	sag	sang
goal	coal	gale	Dale	bag	bang
bigger	bicker	bigger	bidder	hag	hang
tag	tack	rig	rid	hug	hung
bag	back	bug	bud	wig	wing

Additional Notes

The /g/ is mastered at about the same time as /k/ and is seldom misarticulated. Children who have difficulty acquiring /g/ usually substitute /d/ instead. /g/ is the least frequently occurring stop in American English.

FRICATIVES

Fricatives are the largest category of all the consonants. They are all characterized by audible friction. This air turbulence results from the passage of the voiced or voiceless airstream through a narrow opening, usually in the oral cavity. For example, if the narrow opening is between the upper incisors and the lower lip, the fricative /f/ or /v/ will be produced. /s/ and /z/ result from constriction between the tongue tip and the alveolar ridge. If the constriction is between the vocal folds, the consonant /h/ results. There are nine fricative consonants in American English, eight of which occur in cognate pairs: /f/ and /v/, /θ/ and /ð/, /s/ and /z/, and /ʃ/ and /ʒ/. Only the glottal fricative, /h/, has no cognate. Another fricative, /ʍ/, the phoneme in *which* and *quick* is more often pronounced as the glide /w/ in mainstream American English. See the section on Approximants for more information. The fricatives will be presented in cognate pairs, in order of place of articulation, from most anterior to most posterior.

/f/

> IPA symbol: /f/
>
> Cognate: /v/
>
> Description: voiceless labiodental fricative
>
> Key words: fan, offer, leaf
>
> Common spellings: f, ff, ph

/f/ Production

With the velopharyngeal port closed, the lower lip approximates the upper front teeth. Breath is continuously emitted between the teeth and the lower lip as audible friction. The /f/ is usually of greater duration and produced with more force than /v/.

/f/ Words

Initial		Medial		Final		Sequences	
fun	fair	offer	refer	if	beef	fly	soft
feet	fight	before	effort	off	cough	float	sifts
fast	four	coffee	office	wife	tough	free	reflect
five	fine	prophet	coughing	puff	staff	frost	laughs
follow	fort	laughing	profit	laugh	safe	friend	surfed

/f/ Sentences

1. *Frank found fifty* cents in the *field*.
2. *Fran's Friday* classes are *phonetics* and *philosophy*.
3. I saw a whole *field* of *flowers* when I *flew* in yesterday.
4. If you're *free* on *Friday*, let's have *coffee* at the *cafe*.
5. Don't *forget* that *Phil* has moved to a *different office*.

/f/ Contrasts

/f/–/v/		/f/–/θ/		/f/–/p/	
fan	van	Fred	thread	fast	past
fine	vine	fin	thin	fool	pool
feel	veal	free	three	fry	pry

/f/–/v/		/f/–/θ/		/f/–/p/	
surface	service	first	thirst	leaf	leap
proof	prove	reef	wreath	calf	cap
belief	believe	oaf	oath	flee	plea

Additional Notes

/f/ is not a frequently occurring consonant. It is acquired fairly early in development and is seldom misarticulated.

/v/

IPA symbol: /v/

Cognate: /f/

Description: voiced labiodental fricative

Key words: vote, ever, have

Common spelling: v

/v/ Production

/v/ is produced in the same way as /f/ except that the airstream is voiced.

/v/ Words

Initial		Medial		Final		Sequences	
vine	voice	ever	servant	have	believe	obvious	moved
very	vowel	over	fever	gave	weave	advantage	lived
vote	vane	river	diver	live	brave	advent	carved
visit	value	lover	oven	serve	groove	envious	raved
van	vague	aver	proving	move	carve	velvet	served

/v/ Sentences

1. The river divided the village into two halves.
2. We'll need to carve the veal roast when it comes out of the oven.
3. If you divide eleven by five or twelve by seven, the answer will be uneven.
4. Eva bought a new pair of heavy gloves.
5. Vanessa has a lovely voice.
6. Do you vote in the seventeenth or the seventh district?

/v/ Contrasts

/v/–/f/		/v/–/ð/		/v/–/b/		/v/–/w/	
very	fairy	vine	thine	van	ban	vine	wine
vest	fest	van	than	very	berry	vent	went
veal	feel	veil	they'll	vest	best	vet	wet
calve	calf	clover	clothier	serve	Serb	vee	we
prove	proof	lever	leather	savor	saber	vest	west

Additional Notes

The /v/ is mastered fairly late by children, much later than /f/. It is misarticulated with moderate frequency, more often than /f/ but less often than fricatives such as /s/. Spanish speakers may substitute /b/ for /v/ and produce a voiced bilabial fricative in the intervocalic position.

/θ/

> IPA symbol: /θ/
>
> Cognate: /ð/
>
> Description: voiceless (inter)dental fricative
>
> Key words: thumb, nothing, tooth
>
> Common spelling: th

/θ/ Production

The velopharyngeal port is closed, and the sides of the tongue are against the molars. The tip of the tongue, spread wide and thin, approximates the edge of the inner surface of the upper front teeth. The voiceless airstream is continuously emitted between the front teeth and the tongue to create audible friction. The /θ/ is of greater duration and is produced with more force than its cognate, /ð/.

/θ/ Words

Initial		Medial		Final		Sequences	
thin	thaw	anything	nothing	cloth	booth	three	sixth
thank	thud	cathedral	ethics	teeth	growth	threw	month
theme	theft	everything	pathetic	breath	path	threat	length
third	theater	Athens	ether	oath	mouth	booths	earthquake
think	thorn	author	breathy	south	bath	wealthy	width

/θ/ Sentences

1. We'll have to go through Athens coming from north or south.
2. Faith had three candles on her birthday cake.
3. I thought that we needed three tickets for a movie on the fourth.
4. A thief broke into three houses on Thirteenth Street.
5. Measuring length and width is part of your arithmetic assignment.
6. He read through his theme for the third time.

/θ/ Contrasts

/θ/–/ð/		/θ/–/t/		/θ/–/s/	
ether	either	thigh	tie	thumb	some
wreath	wreathe	thin	tin	think	sink
thigh	thy	thick	tick	thaw	saw

/θ/–/ð/		/θ/–/t/		/θ/–/s/	
teeth	teethe	bath	bat	bath	bass
		both	boat	faith	face

Additional Notes

The /θ/ is one of the weakest phonemes acoustically. It is mastered quite late by children and is frequently misarticulated. Substitutions for /θ/ typically are /f/, /t/, and /s/. The /θ/ often creates difficulty for nonnative English speakers because /θ/ occurs in so few languages.

/ð/

Cognate: /θ/

Description: Voiced (inter)dental fricative

Key words: this, weather, breathe

Common spelling: th

/ð/ Production

The /ð/ is produced like the /θ/ except that the airstream is unvoiced. It is of slightly shorter duration and produced with less force than /θ/.

/ð/ Words

Initial		Medial		Final	
the	these	bother	other	soothe	smooth
this	though	weather	lather	bathe	breathe
that	those	rather	feather	writhe	loathe
they	there	either	soothing	tithe	seethe
them	thus	father	mother	teethe	clothe

/ð/ Sentences

1. *The* fea*th*ers bo*th*er *th*em.
2. His fa*th*er and mo*th*er went *th*ere to see *th*em.
3. We can go *th*ere ei*th*er today or tomorrow.
4. Nei*th*er of *th*e girls liked *th*e wea*th*er.
5. I'll need *th*at iron to smoo*th* out *th*e clo*th*ing.
6. They ti*th*e a part of *th*eir income.

/ð/ Contrasts

/ð/–/θ/		/ð/–/d/		/ð/–/v/	
either	ether	then	den	than	van
teethe	teeth	those	doze	that	vat
mouth	mouth	they	day	they'll	veil

/ð/–/θ/		/ð/–/d/		/ð/–/v/	
this	thin	though	dough	either	fever
these	theme	father	fodder	scathe	cave

Additional Notes

Like its cognate /θ/, /ð/ is also among the sounds most frequently in error. Misarticulation may be particularly noticeable because /ð/ occurs in a number of important words such as *the, this, that, then, there (their), them, these,* and *those*. Also like /θ/, /ð/ is one of the last phonemes to be mastered by children. It also causes difficulty for many nonnative English speakers because /ð/ does not occur in a great many languages. Frequent substitutions for /ð/ include /v/, /d/, and /z/, so that *this* might be heard as [dɪs] or [zɪs].

/s/

IPA symbol: /s/

Cognate: /z/

Description: voiceless (lingua-)alveolar fricative

Key words: sun, missing, moss

Common spellings: s, ss, c, x (/k/ + /s/)

/s/ Production

There are two positions commonly used by American English speakers to produce /s/: with the tongue tip up and with the tongue tip down. You can see for yourself: try producing /s/ and noting where your tongue tip is. For most people, the tongue tip is raised, but a sizable minority produce /s/ with the tongue tip lowered. Either position is acceptable as long as a clear /s/ is produced. Both positions, of course, require velopharyngeal closure and a voiceless airstream. In addition, the sides of the tongue rest against the molars for both types. Duration of /s/ is generally longer and breath pressure is greater than for its cognate /z/.

ALVEOLAR /s/: TONGUE TIP UP POSITION. This is the more commonly occurring position for production of /s/. The tongue tip is narrowly grooved and approximates the alveolar ridge just behind the upper incisors. Air flows through the narrow opening created by the tongue tip, alveolar ridge, and closely approximated teeth, producing an audible friction or hissing sound.

DENTAL /s/: TONGUE TIP DOWN POSITION. For this position, the tongue tip approximates the lower incisors near the gum ridge. The front of the tongue is slightly grooved and raised toward the alveolar ridge. Airflow through the narrow opening created by the tongue front, alveolar ridge, and teeth results in the friction or hissing quality of /s/.

/s/ Words

Initial		Medial		Final		Sequences	
see	sun	fasten	missile	us	boss	splash	wasps
sign	sick	lesson	possible	miss	this	spring	mists

Initial		Medial		Final		Sequences	
sour	sip	basin	recent	nice	peace	skin	asks
soup	soap	gasoline	lasso	yes	mice	straw	basket
suit	send	passing	hustle	ice	loss	scream	history

/s/ Sentences

1. *S*am went *s*wimming on*c*e the weather warmed up out*s*ide.
2. *S*ue *s*ketched a *s*mall *s*quare for u*s*.
3. Mi*ss*i*ss*ippi and *S*outh *C*arolina are both *s*outhern *s*tate*s*.
4. Jack'*s* cat*s* *s*ped acro*ss* the *s*treet.
5. Mi*ss* *S*teward is the *s*peaker for the *s*ervice.
6. Le*s* finished the a*ss*ignment from yesterday'*s* hi*s*tory le*ss*on.

/s/ Contrasts

/s/–/z/		/s/–/θ/		/s/–/ʃ/	
see	z	sin	thin	sue	shoe
sue	zoo	sank	thank	sign	shine
fleece	flees	seem	theme	fasten	fashion
bus	buzz	gross	growth	mass	mash
racer	razor	face	faith	Swiss	swish

Additional Notes

The /s/ is one of the most frequently occurring American English consonant sounds as well as one of the most frequently misarticulated consonants. Consequently, a problem with /s/ (**lisp**) can be quite disruptive to speech understandability. The /θ/ is a frequent substitution for /s/, so that *s*un may be produced as [θ ʌ n]. Dentition issues can play a role in poor /s/ production; for example, dentures in an older adult may lend a whistling quality to /s/. The loss of central incisors by children between ages 5 and 7 frequently results in a temporary lisp. High-frequency hearing loss is also associated with misarticulation of /s/.

/z/

IPA symbol: /z/

Cognate: /s/

Description: voiced (lingua-)alveolar fricative

Key words: zoo, razor, size

Common spellings: z, zz, s

/z/ Production

Like /s/, there are two prevalent formations for /z/ production, with tongue tip up more often used. These formations are exactly like those for /s/ with one exception: the airstream is voiced. Duration and breath pressure for /z/ are usually less than for its cognate /s/.

/z/ Words

Initial		Medial		Final		Sequences
zoo	zebra	easy	visit	buzz	is	songs
zipper	zinc	dozen	nozzle	jazz	was	webs
zone	Zen	music	dizzy	these	breeze	gives
zero	zodiac	puzzle	dozing	use	those	adds
zest	xylophone	busy	weasel	nose	lose	eggs

/z/ Sentences

1. The weasel's eyes were closed.
2. Our neighbors will be visiting their relatives in Arizona.
3. Jan's recipe calls for a dozen eggs.
4. The jazz musician dazzled the audience.
5. Point the nozzle on the hose toward the flowers.
6. The girls worked busily on the puzzle.

/z/ Contrasts

/z/–/s/		/z/–/ð/		/z/–/ʒ/	
zeal	seal	bays	bathe	bays	beige
Zack	sack	breeze	breathe	lows	loge
zone	sewn	close	clothe	rues	rouge
fleas	fleece	seas	seethe	Caesar	seizure
lose	loose	tease	teethe	glazer	glazier

Additional Notes

The /z/, like its cognate /s/, is one of the last consonants mastered by children. It is also one of the most frequently misarticulated sounds, most often replaced by /ð/. Some speakers from Europe may substitute /s/ for /z/ as well.

/ʃ/

IPA symbol: /ʃ/

Cognate: /ʒ/

Description: voiceless (lingua-)palatal fricative

Key words: shoe, wishing, wash

Common spellings: sh, s

/ʃ/ Production

The velopharyngeal port is closed, and a voiceless airstream is used throughout production. The sides of the tongue are against the upper molars, and the broad front surface of the tongue is raised toward the palate just behind the alveolar ridge. This forms a central opening that is slightly broader and farther back than for /s/ production. The voiceless airstream is directed continuously through and against the slightly open front teeth to produce audible friction. The lips are usually slightly rounded and protruded, similar to the position for /ʊ/.

/ʃ/ Words

Initial		Medial		Final		Sequences
sheep	shine	fashion	wishes	mash	radish	shrimp
chic	shut	bushel	fishing	mesh	English	shrink
shall	shake	ashamed	rushing	wish	splash	washed
shield	show	ocean	fuchsia	fresh	crush	fished
ship	shade	assure	nation	relish	push	insurance

/ʃ/ Sentences

1. *She shook the shirt after washing and drying it.*
2. *Facial expressions should show emotion.*
3. *That new fashion looks very chic on Michelle.*
4. *Shelley shut the door and then rushed off.*
5. *We'll take an ocean-going ship for our vacation.*
6. *Sheldon is shining shoes.*

/ʃ/ Contrasts

/ʃ/–/ʒ/		/ʃ/–/s/		/ʃ/–/tʃ/	
glacier	glazier	sheet	seat	shad	Chad
Aleutian	allusion	shoe	sue	chic	cheek
assure	azure	she	see	ship	chip
leash	liege	lashes	lasses	marsh	march
dilution	delusion	gash	gas	bush	butch

Additional Notes

The /ʃ/ is another one of the consonants that is frequently in error. The /s/ is a common substitution for /ʃ/, so that *shoe* may be heard as [s u]. The /ʃ/ may also be affected if English is a speaker's second language; for example, Spanish speakers may substitute /tʃ/ for /ʃ/. Further details regarding dialectic variation may be found in Chapter 8.

/ʒ/

IPA symbol: /ʒ/

Cognate: /ʃ/

Description: voiced (lingua-)palatal fricative

Key words: measure, corsage

Common spellings: variable (see examples)

/ʒ/ Production

The velopharyngeal port is closed, and the airstream is voiced throughout production. Formation of /ʒ/ is just like that for /ʃ/ except that the airstream is voiced.

/ʒ/ Words

/ʒ/ occurs only in the medial and final positions of words in English.

Medial		Final	
vision	aphasia	beige	corsage
usual	treasure	loge	garage
casual	occasion	rouge	prestige
measure	seizure	montage	camouflage
lesion	regime	collage	triage

/ʒ/ Sentences

1. Occasionally, decisions can lead to confusion.
2. The collision and explosion caused a lesion that affected his vision.
3. She measured the beige garage.
4. The special occasion gave him great pleasure.
5. We'll have to be careful about the division of the treasure.
6. Her role in the regime gave her great prestige.

/ʒ/ Contrasts

/ʒ/–/ʃ/		/ʒ/–/ʤ/	
glazier	glacier	pleasure	pledger
vision	vicious	lesion	legion
measure	mesh	vision	pigeon
occasion	vacation	rouge	huge
azure	assure	prestige	vestige

Additional Notes

The /ʒ/ is one of the last consonants to be developed and mastered by children. It is also one of the least frequently occurring consonants in English. In some American English dialects, /ʒ/ may be replaced by /ʤ/ for certain words. For example, garage might be pronounced as [gəraʒ] or [gəraʤ].

/h/

IPA symbol: /h/

Cognate: none

Description: voiceless glottal fricative

Key words: he, ahead

Common spellings: h, wh

/h/ Production

The velopharyngeal port is closed. The vocal folds are slightly adducted, creating a constriction through which the voiceless airstream is forced. This results in the friction sound recognized as /h/. Because /h/ is formed at the glottis, the oral cavity structures are free to assume any of the vowel positions that follow /h/.

/h/ Words

/h/ occurs only in the prevocalic and intervocalic positions in English.

Initial		Medial	
he	high	ahead	unhook
his	how	behind	mahogany
her	hat	perhaps	anyhow
hoe	home	rehearse	behold
who	hook	mohair	behave

/h/ Sentences

1. *H*ank left *h*is *h*at at *h*ome.
2. Per*h*aps we should re*h*earse the *h*igh parts again.
3. Does *H*olly want to go a*h*ead or follow be*h*ind?
4. *Wh*o *h*as a *h*ouse on the *h*ighway?
5. The *h*air on *h*is *h*ead *h*ad turned gray.
6. *H*elen *h*as to learn *h*ow to be*h*ave.

/h/ Contrasts

/h/–/ /		/h/–/θ/	
heat	eat	hatch	thatch
hit	it	high	thigh
hate	ate	hum	thumb
hair	air	heard	third
head	Ed	hug	thug

Additional Notes

The /h/ is one of the earliest sounds mastered by children; consequently, complete omission of /h/ in words, even in young children, may indicate a problem. The /h/ is subject to some voicing when it occurs between voiced phonemes. We will discuss this further in Chapter 6.

AFFRICATES

There are only two affricates in American English, the cognates /tʃ/ and /ʤ/ (as in *chair* and *jump,* respectively). Affricates share characteristics of both stops and fricatives in their manner of formation. Consequently, their symbols are actually a combination of those you already know. Each is still one phoneme, however, because of the coarticulation involved. The single phoneme is also indicated by the touching of the component symbols in transcription for each affricate.

For both American English affricates, the oral airstream is briefly interrupted or stopped (like a stop), then released with friction (like a fricative). The stop and the fricative sound are smoothly blended as one phoneme.

/tʃ/

IPA symbol: /tʃ/

Cognate: /ʤ/

Description: voiceless (lingua-)palatal affricate

Key words: chair, teacher, watch

Common spellings: ch, tch

/tʃ/ Production

The velopharyngeal port is closed, and the sides of the tongue approximate the upper molars. The tongue tip closes on or just behind the alveolar ridge, and the voiceless airstream is held and compressed in the oral cavity. Following this air compression, the air is forced through a narrow constriction formed by the tongue and palate to complete the /ʃ/ phase of /tʃ/. The entire phoneme is produced on a single impulse of breath.

/tʃ/ Words

Initial		Medial		Final	
chain	chair	kitchen	bachelor	watch	each
choose	cheese	nature	natural	much	such
change	chase	virtue	catcher	church	reach
chin	children	matches	preacher	coach	which
chilled	chapter	richest	peaches	beach	latch

/tʃ/ Sentences

1. The *ch*ildren had pea*ch*es at lun*ch*.
2. *Ch*ad *ch*ose *ch*erry *ch*eesecake.
3. We wa*tch*ed them mar*ch* toward the bea*ch*.
4. *Ch*et found ma*tch*es in the ki*tch*en.
5. *Ch*ocolate *ch*ess pie is great for lun*ch*.
6. Ea*ch* *ch*apter includes questions to *ch*eck your understanding.

/tʃ/ Contrasts

/tʃ/–/dʒ/		/tʃ/–/ʃ/		/tʃ/–/t/	
chain	Jane	chair	share	chime	time
cheep	jeep	chin	shin	chew	two
chunk	junk	matching	mashing	chin	tin
batches	badges	hutch	hush	batch	bat
lunch	lunge	much	mush	kitchen	kitten

Additional Notes

The /tʃ/ also is one of the consonants most likely to be misarticulated. The /ʃ/ is often substituted for /tʃ/ in typical misarticulations, resulting in words like *chest* being produced as [ʃ ɛ s t]. The /tʃ/ may also be misarticulated by some nonnative English speakers.

/dʒ/

IPA symbol: /dʒ/

Cognate: /tʃ/

Description: voiced (lingua-)palatal affricate

Key words: jump, badger, edge

Common spellings: j, dg(e)

/dʒ/ Production

The /dʒ/ is produced in the same way as /tʃ/ except for use of a voiced airstream.

/dʒ/ Words

Initial		Medial		Final	
jam	giant	lodges	gradual	age	village
jaw	gem	badger	merger	edge	bridge
joy	gentle	codger	agent	gauge	cottage
jelly	gene	agitate	ridges	ledge	college
Jim	general	ginger	magic	urge	strange

/dʒ/ Sentences

1. The judge and jury gauged the logic of his argument.
2. You can buy jam and jelly from Janis.
3. Madge won't budge from the ledge.
4. Our fiscal agent will review the ledger for the general store.
5. The soldier, sargeant, and major were all outranked by the general.
6. Jess jammed all the junk in the garbage can.

/ʤ/ Contrasts

/ʤ/ – /ʧ/		/ʤ/ – /j/		/ʤ/ – /dz/	
jeer	cheer	jam	yam	budge	buds
jump	chump	jeer	year	rage	raids
age	H	juice	use	siege	seeds
gin	chin	gel	yell	wage	wades
joke	choke	jet	yet	age	aids

Additional Notes

Like its cognate /ʧ/, /ʤ/ is one of the most frequently misarticulated sounds and one of the last mastered by children. Typically, a /ʃ/ is substituted for /ʧ/ when this phoneme is misarticulated. The /ʧ/ occurs more frequently than /ʤ/ but is nevertheless a very low occurrence consonant. Correct articulation may pose problems for some speakers of English as a second language.

Nasals

The three nasal resonant consonants of American English are /m/, /n/, and /ŋ/. They are produced by alteration of the cavities of the vocal tract (as are approximants, which follow in the next section). The nasals differ from consonants with oral airflow in one particularly important way: the velopharyngeal port is open, permitting open resonation of the voiced airstream in the nasal cavity. At the same time, the oral cavity is completely closed off at some point, forcing the airflow through the nasal cavity. For /m/ production, the resonating cavity consists of the open nasal cavity and the oral cavity occluded at the lips. The resonating space for /ŋ/ is smaller, with oral closure at the alveolar ridge. The resonating space for /n/ uses even less oral cavity space because closure is made with the back of the tongue and the velum. Discrimination among the nasals usually does not cause difficulty except for /n/ and /ŋ/ in certain contexts. Also, /n/ is sometimes substituted for /ŋ/ in rapid speech and in some dialects (e.g., *runnin'* for *running*).

/m/

IPA symbol: /m/

Description: (voiced) bilabial nasal

Key words: my, coming, team

Common spellings: m, mm

/m/ Production

The lips are closed, and the velopharyngeal port is open. The voiced airstream is directed out through the nasal cavity and the nostrils. The tongue lies flat in the mouth or is prepared for the following vowel. The teeth are slightly open.

/m/ Words

Initial		Medial		Final		Sequences	
me	men	summer	coming	am	term	small	jump
may	much	hammer	remind	whom	time	smile	hums
meat	might	animal	among	lamb	diaphragm	lamp	somewhere
miss	mat	family	blooming	hymn	team	blimp	Christmas
more	moon	America	humid	plum	roam	smell	stormed
must	mark	calming	combing	hum	column	chums	hemmed

/m/ Sentences

1. Remember them at Christmas in December.
2. Mark groomed the lamb for the farm competition.
3. I'm hoping to have more time off next summer.
4. Be on time or you'll miss the opening hymn.
5. That little Michael is really a motor mouth.
6. Use the camera to get that image on film.

/m/ Contrasts

/m/–/b/		/m/–/n/		/m/–/ŋ/	
mite	bite	me	knee	ham	hang
mean	bean	mine	nine	hum	hung
rum	rub	hem	hen	swim	swing
come	cub	ram	ran	Sam	sang
lambs	labs	terms	turns	Kim	king

Additional Notes

The /m/ is one of the first sounds mastered by children and is seldom misarticulated. It is also one of the most frequently occurring sounds in English.

/n/

IPA symbol: /n/

Description: (voiced) alveolar nasal

Key words: no, many, green

Common spellings: n, nn

/n/ Production

Production of /n/ is just like that of /m/ except that oral closure is made with the tip of the tongue against the alveolar ridge and the sides of the tongue against the upper molars.

/n/ Words

Initial		Medial		Final		Sequences	
not	gnat	funny	banana	can	ripen	snail	hunt
knife	north	many	peanut	align	cotton	snow	hind
new	gnarled	any	enemy	sign	kitten	snake	bald
know	nap	tiny	annotate	inn	on	under	pint
name	nice	Annie	Dennis	been	seen	Indiana	pines

/n/ Sentences

1. I'll need a knife to spread this peanut butter.
2. Do you know the name of the new man?
3. The snow landed gently on the pine trees.
4. The new movie is playing down at the big screen cinema.
5. There are seven candidates running for that office right now.
6. Jane put down the knife after she finished cutting the cake.

/n/ Contrasts

/n/–/d/		/n/–/m/		/n/–/ŋ/	
need	deed	Nate	mate	ban	bang
no	doe	night	might	fan	fang
owner	odor	turns	terms	pin	ping
bin	bid	dine	dime	thin	thing
can	cad	own	ohm	sun	sung

Additional Notes

Like /m/, /n/ is one of the first sounds mastered by children and is seldom misarticulated. In addition, /n/ is the most frequently occurring consonant in English.

/ŋ/

IPA symbol: /ŋ/

Description: (voiced) velar nasal

Key words: song, ringer

Common spellings: ng, n

/ŋ/ Production

The /ŋ/ is produced like /n/ except that oral cavity closure is made by the back of the tongue against the front part of the velum or back part of the palate. Tongue pressure at the velum is less than for /k/ or /g/.

/ŋ/ Words

/ŋ/ does not occur in the initial position in English.

Medial		Final		Sequences	
singer	hanger	tongue	along	linger	longer
ringer	singing	sang	lung	anger	thanks
hanging	swinger	running	working	banked	rings
pinging	winging	among	string	think	younger
stinger	zinger	meaning	long	kangaroo	longed

/ŋ/ Sentences

1. We'll lengthen the sleeves to make them long enough for the singer.
2. Frank needs a drink of water after working so hard.
3. Doing things like running will help you live longer.
4. Among the singers, the youngest one was the strongest performer.
5. Is anyone bringing drinks for the party?
6. The mockingbird sang and then spread its wings to fly away.

/ŋ/ Contrasts

/ŋ/–/g/		/ŋ/–/n/		/ŋ/–/m/	
wing	wig	stung	stun	hung	hum
tongue	tug	long	lawn	ding	dim
longing	logging	wing	win	clang	clam
bang	bag	tongue	ton	sung	sum
longed	logged	hung	Hun	hanger	hammer

Additional Notes

The /ŋ/ is also mastered early by children (though later than /m/ and /n/). It is seldom misarticulated. In informal speech, /n/ often replaces /ŋ/ in words such as *running* ([rʌnɪn]) and *jumping* ([ʤʌmpɪn]).

APPROXIMANTS/ORAL RESONANT CONSONANTS

This manner category encompasses four phonemes: /j/ (as in *yes*), /w/ (*wing*), /l/ (*lend*), and /ɹ/ (*rug*). They are characterized by alterations of the resonating cavities for their distinctive identities. The four consonants are often subdivided into two, smaller classes: **glides** (/w/ and /j/, also sometimes referred to as **semivowels**) and **liquids** (/l/ and /ɹ/).

/w/

IPA symbol: /w/

Description: (voiced) (lingua-)velar bilabial glide

Key words: we, away

Common spellings: w, wh

/w/ Production

With the velopharyngeal port closed, the lips are rounded (labial placement) for an opening slightly smaller than for the vowel /u/. At the same time, the tongue is elevated (velar placement) in the back of the mouth as for /u/. The voiced airstream is directed into the oral cavity, and the articulators move or "glide" from this initial posture into the position of the vowel that must follow the /w/. The /w/ is of short duration and is always released into a vowel.

Some speakers differentiate between the /w/ in *witch* and the ʍ in *which*. However, most mainstream American English speakers use /w/ for both forms. We will follow that practice in this section.

/w/ Words

Initial		Medial		Sequences	
we	wash	away	rewind	twin	twist
way	weed	freeway	seaweed	queen	quick
were	won	anyone	byway	Gwen	swell
wet	one	forward	tower	sweet	sweater
wood	would	reward	otherwise	twilight	quest

/w/ Sentences

1. *We went wading in the water anyway.*
2. *Wes went away last week.*
3. *Gwen always goes away for the winter.*
4. *Dwight could see the woods from his west window.*
5. *Will prefers our warm windy weather to the cold and snow of winter.*
6. *Did she win by moving forward or backward?*

/w/ Contrasts

/w/–/l/		/w/–/r/		/w/–/v/	
wed	led	white	right	we	vee
weed	lead	when	wren	wary	vary
wake	lake	wind	rind	wet	vet
wise	lies	wake	rake	went	vent
wick	lick	west	rest	wail	vale

Additional Notes

The /w/ is mastered very early by children and is seldom misarticulated. It is often substituted for /l/ and /ɹ/ in children's early speech development. Thus, *lamp* might be produced as [w æ m p] and *ring* as [w ɪ ŋ].

/j/

IPA symbol: /j/

Description: (voiced)(lingua-)palatal glide

Key words: you, bayou

Common Spelling: y

/j/ Production

The velopharyngeal port is closed, and the tip of the tongue is positioned behind the lower front teeth. The front of the tongue is raised high toward the palate. The voiced airstream is directed through the oral cavity for a brief period as the tongue and lips assume the position for the following vowel. The space between the tongue and the palate is similar to that for /i/. Duration of /j/ is short, and it is always released into a vowel.

/j/ Words

Initial		Medial		Sequences	
yard	young	loyal	beyond	few	music
year	yes	bayou	rayon	cute	onion
yet	yellow	royal	hallelujah	barnyard	minion
yolk	use	foyer	higher	million	muse
yarn	unit	voyage		pupil	canyon

/j/ Sentences

1. William went to see the Grand Canyon last year.
2. Yesterday the youngsters were companions.
3. Are you sure that you're going to say yes?
4. The pupils went beyond the yellow line.
5. Few of the musicians liked the new music composition.
6. The young family came from New York.

/j/ Contrasts

/j/–/w/		/j/–/ɹ/		/j/–/ʤ/	
yet	wet	yam	am	yam	jam
yoke	woke	year	ear	yell	jell
yield	wield	yearn	earn	yet	jet
yell	well	beauty	booty	yak	Jack
yes	Wes	cute	coot	year	jeer

Additional Notes

Some phoneticians consider /j/ as a diphthong when it is released into /u/, for example, /ju/ in *cute,* and *few.* We will treat it as part of a consonant sequence in this book. The /j/ is acquired fairly early and is seldom misarticulated. It is not a frequently occurring sound.

/l/

IPA symbol: /l/

Description: (voiced) (lingua-)alveolar liquid

Key words: lamp, balloon, bell

Common spellings: l, ll, le

/l/ Description

The velopharyngeal port is closed, and the airstream is voiced throughout production. There are actually two articulatory positions for /l/, with use depending on the position (prevocalic, postvocalic) of the consonant in a word. For prevocalic /l/, the tongue tip closes with slight pressure against the alveolar ridge, with an opening on both sides. This allows the voiced airstream to escape laterally around the tongue and out the oral cavity. (Hence, **lateral phoneme** is another term that is used to describe /l/.) When /l/ occurs in the postvocalic position, the back of the tongue is also raised toward the velum, in addition to the tongue tip elevation. For prevocalic /l/, the tongue tip leaves the alveolar ridge to form the next phoneme. The tongue tip stays at the alveolar ridge for postvocalic /l/.

/l/ Words

Initial		Medial		Final		Sequences	
lay	loose	yellow	hollow	oil	bell	plant	flower
leaf	lunch	tulip	dollar	all	fall	glass	clock
low	lamb	eleven	fellow	mill	school	slide	glee
like	leg	lily	jelly	hole	tell	climb	sled
lion	lift	along	teller	motel	fail	aglow	onslaught

/l/ Sentences

1. *L*ou *l*iked to have *l*unch after his *l*esson.
2. There were ye*ll*ow tu*l*ips b*l*ooming a*ll* over the hi*ll*side.
3. The peop*l*e took a seat at the midd*l*e tab*l*e.
4. They did *l*eg *l*ifts as part of the ba*ll*et c*l*ass.
5. Map*l*e *l*eaves fa*ll* off the trees in the fa*ll* months.

/l/ Contrasts

/l/–/w/		/l/–/r/		/l/–/n/	
let	wet	lane	rain	line	nine
Lou	woo	lair	rare	lead	need
line	wine	load	road	low	no
lack	whack	play	prey	slow	snow
Lee's	wheeze	Clyde	cried	tell	ten

Additional Notes

The /l/ is mastered late by children. It is often replaced by a /w/ (or sometimes a /j/) in early speech development, so that *lamp* may be produced as [wæmp] or [jæmp]. It is one of the sounds most frequently misarticulated, though not as often as /s/. Speakers of English Asian dialect may confuse /l/ and /r/. See Chapter 8 for further information.

/ɹ/

IPA symbol: /ɹ/

Description: (voiced) (lingua-)palatal liquid

Key words: run, caring, car

Common spellings: r, rr

/ɹ/ Production

The /ɹ/ can be produced in several different ways, even by the same speaker. All productions require velopharyngeal closure and a voiced airstream. Regardless of specific position, the key to /ɹ/ production is that the tongue is held high in the oral cavity but does not touch the roof of the mouth. This allows a central flow of air from the oral cavity (as opposed to the lateral airflow of /l/). Three positions have been described.

TONGUE TIP UP POSITION   The sides of the tongue are against the upper molars. The tongue tip is raised toward the palate just behind the alveolar ridge but does not make contact with it. The voiced airstream escapes between the tongue and the palato-alveolar area, out of the oral cavity. The lips may be slightly protruded in a position similar to /ʊ/, but they usually take the position of the following vowel. For example, for the /ɹ/ in *rain,* the lips are spread for [eɪ], but in *room,* the lips are rounded in anticipation of the [u]. (You can see this for yourself if you say the two words while looking in a mirror.)

RETROFLEX POSITION   This is a variation of the tongue tip up position. It is produced in the same way except that the tongue tip is curled up and back.

TONGUE TIP DOWN POSITION   The sides of the tongue are against the upper molars. The front of the tongue is raised toward the palate, with the tip neutral or pointing downward.

/ɹ/ Words

Postvocalic /ɹ/ is transcribed as a consonant, rather than as part of a centering diphthong, in this section and throughout the remainder of the book.

Initial		Medial		Final		Sequences	
ran	write	very	marry	car	or	bring	bright
red	wrist	around	terrible	air	dear	drain	draw
rub	rhyme	orange	berry	four	chair	pray	pride
rake	right	story	arrow	near	are	travel	trust
rose	roam	carrot	sorry	fire	dare	straw	street
rock	wren	carry	eerie	hair	bar	tread	toothbrush

/ɹ/ Sentences

1. I need three more chairs for the dining room.
2. There was a terrible rainstorm around four o'clock on Friday.
3. Sarah raked the grass after she mowed it.
4. Rob told Rita the story about the car race.
5. Rich needs more oregano for the rigatoni dish he's preparing.

/ɹ/ Contrasts

/ɹ/–/w/		/ɹ/–/l/		/ɹ/–/ɝ/ or /ɚ/	
rip	whip	rest	lest	train	terrain
rich	witch	red	led	bray	beret
run	one	Rick	lick	dress	duress
raid	wade	room	loom	crest	caressed
rock	wok	ride	lied	broke	baroque
trig	twig	brink	blink	throw	thorough
trice	twice	crone	clone	creed	curried
tryst	twist	cram	clam	crowed	corrode

Additional Notes

The /ɹ/ is acquired later in speech development and is one of the sounds most frequently in error. Substitution of /w/ for /ɹ/ is common in early childhood. The /ɹ/ is also subject to dialectic variation depending on the type of English (e.g., British and Hispanic) and region of the United States. For example, intervocalic /ɹ/ is trilled in British English, making words like *very* sound like [vɛdi]. In New England and Southern English, the postvocalic /ɹ/ may be omitted or replaced by a vowel, for example, resulting in *here* being produced as [hijə] or *park* being produced as [pɑk]. Further information on multicultural speech variations will be found in Chapter 8.

The consonant /ɹ/ differs from the **rhotic** vowels /ɝ/ and /ɚ/ in three ways: (1) it is shorter in duration, (2) it never constitutes a syllable, and (3) movement is away from the /ɹ/ position (as opposed to the rhotic vowels' movement toward the /ɹ/ position).

REVIEW VOCABULARY

abutting consonants   two or more adjacent consonants that cross a syllable boundary.

affricate   consonant produced by release of a stop into a fricative position as a single speech sound. English affricate consonants are /ʧ/ and /ʤ/.

approximant   consonant with characteristics of both vowels and consonants, produced with less constriction than stops, fricatives, and affricates.

aspiration   audible release of breath, as with the [p] in *pot*.

coarticulation   influence of one speech sound on the adjacent sound in connected speech.

consonant   phoneme used marginally with a vowel to constitute a syllable; characterized by narrowing or blockage of the airstream.

consonant blend   consonant sequence in which two or more adjacent consonants occur within the same syllable.

consonant sequence   two or more adjacent consonants within or across a syllable boundary.

fricative   phoneme produced with audible friction as a result of narrowing of the vocal tract at some point. English fricative consonants are /f/ /v/ /θ/, /ð/, /s/, /z/, /ʃ,/ /ʒ/, and /h/.

glide   consonant produced by an initial narrowing of the vocal tract followed by transition into the following vowel. English glides are /j/ and /w/.

intervocalic consonant   singleton consonant separating two vowels in a word.

lateral phoneme   a consonant phoneme in which the voiced airstream escapes around the sides of the tongue. The English lateral is /l/. See Liquid.

liquid   consonant phonemes produced with the tongue acting as an obstacle to the outgoing voiced airstream. English liquids are /ɹ/ and /l/.

lisp   problem with correct production of /s/.

manner of articulation   refers to the way the voiced or voiceless airstream is modified to produce different types of consonants (e.g., stops and fricatives).

nasal   consonant phonemes produced with lowering of the soft palate and closure within the oral cavity, allowing for a nasal airflow of the voiced airstream. English nasals are /m/, /n/, and /ŋ/.

oral resonant   consonant produced with voiced oral airflow; includes glides, liquids, and nasals.

plosive   see Aspiration.

postvocalic consonant   singleton consonant following a vowel.

prevocalic consonant   singleton consonant preceding a vowel.

retroflex   a bending backward of the tongue, especially applied to the tongue position for retroflex /r/.

rhotic   adjective referring to positioning or influence of /ɹ/.

semivowel   see Glide.

singleton consonant   a consonant with no other consonants immediately adjacent to it.

stop   consonant phoneme produced with closure or stopping of the airstream; air may or may not be released. English stops are /p/, /b/, /t/, /d/, /k/, and /g/.

EXERCISES

1. Identify the boldfaced consonants in the following words with regard to position and makeup (singleton or sequence).

	Position	Singleton/Sequence
a.	[r eɪ z ɚ]	
b.	[b æ sk ə t]	
c.	[t u θ b r ʌ ʃ]	
d.	[b ɝ d h aʊ s]	
e.	[ʧ ɛ r]	
f.	[l æ m p]	
g.	[b l ɑ k s]	

2. Write the IPA symbol that matches each of the following brief descriptions:
   a. Bilabial nasal:
   b. Voiceless alveolar stop:
   c. Voiceless palatal fricative:
   d. Voiced velar stop:
   e. Voiceless (inter)dental fricative:
   f. Palatal glide:
   g. Voiceless labiodental fricative:
   h. Voiceless palatal affricate:
   i. Bilabial-velar glide:
   j. Voiced (inter)dental fricative:
   k. Voiced alveolar fricative:
   l. Velar nasal:
   m. Voiced palatal fricative:
   n. Voiced labiodental fricative:
   o. Voiced bilabial stop:
   p. Alveolar liquid:
   q. Voiceless bilabial stop:
   r. Voiceless glottal fricative:
   s. Alveolar nasal:
   t. Voiced alveolar stop:
   u. Voiceless velar stop:
   v. Voiced palatal affricate:
   w. Palatal liquid:

3. List the cognate for each of the following:
   a. /p/_____   b. /z/_____   c. /ʤ/_____   d. /f/_____
   e. /t/_____   f. /ʒ/_____   g. /θ/_____   h. /k/_____

4. List all the consonants included in each group described below:
   a. Voiced alveolar consonants:
   b. Palatal consonants:
   c. Voiced stop consonants:
   d. Voiceless fricative consonants:
   e. Nasal consonants:

    f.   Voiced velar consonants:

    g.   Labial consonants:

    h.   Voiced affricate:

5. For each group of phonemes listed, indicate the characteristic(s) they share in common, for example, /b w v/: voiced, labial place of articulation.

    a.   /s l n d/

    b.   /ʤ ʒ/

    c.   /r l/

    d.   /r ʒ ʧ j/

    e.   /k ŋ/

    f.   /z t d/

    g.   /g d ð n ʒ/

    h.   /p b w/

CHAPTER 6

CONNECTED SPEECH: SEGMENTAL AND SUPRASEGMENTAL EFFECTS

INFLUENCES OF CONTEXT: COARTICULATION
SPEECH RHYTHM AND SUPRASEGMENTAL FEATURES
REVIEW VOCABULARY
EXERCISES

INFLUENCES OF CONTEXT: COARTICULATION

Up to this point, we have analyzed speech in terms of its **segmental** (phoneme) components and then, only in a somewhat artificial way. As you know, we have described each phoneme as a segment with an individualized description for the formation of each. Our intent was to provide a fundamental understanding of the units that make up connected speech. You had many terms and symbols to learn, and they were best learned as individual entities, one at a time. If you recall, however, we told you earlier that speech really does not occur in distinctly separate segments. In normal (real, connected) speech, phonemes do not follow each other the way beads on a string do. That is, you do not produce a word or phrase by simply producing an individual phoneme, then moving on to the next phoneme, and so on. Instead, there is a constant, overlapping effect of the movements of the articulators so that each phoneme's production overlaps and is therefore influenced by the ones surrounding it. There is a term to refer to this influence of adjoining sounds on each other: **coarticulation.** Coarticulation means that the vocal tract can take more than one position at the same time so that connected speech occurs as a continuous flow, rather than as a series of individually produced phonemes. Coarticulation means that the movements of the articulators will be efficient and makes connected speech easier to produce. Before we discuss the different types of coarticulatory effects, we will start with a few examples that you can try for yourself.

First, look in a mirror and say these two words in succession: /ʃi/ and /ʃu/. Notice the position of your lips as you produce the /ʃ/ each time. You should notice that your lips are spread for /ʃ/ production in *she* but rounded for the /ʃ/ in *shoe*. The actual identity of the consonant /ʃ/ is not changed, but its manner of formation differs slightly depending on the vowel that follows it. This is one example of coarticulation. In this example, the lip rounding (an articulatory feature of the vowel [u]) is coarticulated with the consonant [ʃ].

Next, try saying this phrase quickly three times: *so easy*. Pay careful attention to the sound that appears between /oʊ/ and /i/. Did you notice a /w/ "sneaking in" so that *easy* sounded a little like *wheezy*? In this case, coarticulation has produced an additional or intrusive sound as the articulators transition from the /oʊ/ position to the /i/ position. (See Addition/Epenthesis later in this chapter.) The appearance of /w/ should not be too surprising because the transition involved is from a rounded vowel position ([oʊ]) to a "spread" vowel ([i]). The movement involved is very much like the /w/ formation described in Chapter 5. You may also notice /w/ intrusion due to coarticulation in phrases such as *to each* [tuwitʃ] and *to a* [tuwə].

The coarticulation effects discussed in this chapter are among the most commonly occurring in American English. You will find exercises at the end of this chapter to help you understand these effects. For some of the effects, you will also find exercises in Chapters 11–15 in the workbook to help you learn these aspects of narrow transcription.

DURATION

EFFECTS ON VOWELS

You have probably already noticed that phonemes naturally vary in duration; for example, vowels are longer in duration than stops. In connected speech, the length of vowel sounds is also influenced by the manner of articulation of the consonant that follows them. Vowels typically are shorter before a stop consonant or affricate than before a fricative or resonant consonant. Try saying these word pairs, and note the difference in vowel duration for each pair member:

> ease [iz]——eat [it]   if [ɪf]——it [ɪt]
> tame [teɪm]——take [teɪk]   us [ʌs]——up [ʌp]

Vowel duration may also be affected by the voicing of the consonant that follows it in connected speech. A vowel will have shorter duration before a voiceless stop or affricate than before its voiced counterpart, made in the same position. Compare the difference in vowel duration in the following pairs of words:

> edge [ɛdʒ]——etch [ɛtʃ]   sub [sʌb]——sup [sʌp]
> ad [æd]——at [æt]   bag [bæg]——back [bæk]
> lab [læb]——lap [læp]   sued [sud]——suit [sut]

In the following examples, notice how vowel duration differs in each set of words as a result of manner and voicing of the following consonant (note that the place of articulation is the same for each word set):

> ad [æd]——an [æn]——at [æt]
> cub [kʌb]——come [kʌm]——cup [kʌp]
> lug [lʌg]——lung [lʌŋ]——luck [lʌk]

EFFECTS ON CONSONANTS

In the previous examples, it was not necessary to use any narrow transcription symbol to indicate the difference in vowel duration that resulted from coarticulation. However, there are several symbols that are used to indicate durational changes in consonant (and sometimes vowel) articulation.

The first example requiring a narrow transcription symbol occurs when the same consonant is produced at the end of one word and the beginning of another. Contrast the duration of /m/ in these expressions: *summon* (/m/ articulated as one nasal consonant) and *some more* (/m/ prolonged). In expressions of the second type (same consonant ending a word and beginning the following word), the two consonants will be produced as one sound, but the duration is usually extended. This difference is indicated in narrow transcription with the symbol [:] (which looks like a colon and follows the phoneme with increased length):

summon [sʌmən]	some men [sʌm:ɛn]
falling [fɔlɪŋ]	fall line [fɔl:aɪn]
topping [tɑpɪŋ]	top pair [tɑp:ɛr]

SYLLABIC CONSONANTS   Another characteristic of connected speech affects resonant consonants (specifically /m/, /n/, and /l/). They may be increased in duration to actually take the role of a syllable nucleus (vowel) under certain conditions. If one of these consonants occurs in the postvocalic position immediately after a consonant with the same position, the /ə/ may be omitted in favor of lengthening the /m/, /n/, or /l/. Syllabic consonants are marked by the diacritic []. Try saying the following words, first with the [ə] and then with a syllabic consonant for the syllable nucleus.

ridden	[rɪdən]	[rɪdn̩]
huddle	[hʌdəl]	[hʌdl̩]
blossom	[blɑsəm]	[blɑsm̩]

Did you notice how much more "natural" the words with syllabic consonants sounded? You will recognize this effect even more in the following examples of phrases that include syllabic consonants (and accompanying consonant deletion):

stop them	[stɑpðɛm]	[stɑpm̩]
you and me	[juændmi]	[jun̩mi]
it will do	[ɪtwɪldu]	[ɪdl̩du]

You will find more examples of these coarticulation effects at the end of this chapter and also in the workbook in Chapter 11.

ASPIRATION OF STOPS

You learned in Chapter 5 that the release (aspiration) phase of stops is optional. In mainstream American English, prevocalic voiceless stops are always audibly aspirated or released. Singleton postvocalic stops and singleton stops that occur at the ends of utterances, however, are often not released. Alternatively, they may be released so gently that audible aspiration is unnoticeable. Audible stop aspiration is transcribed using the diacritic marking ['] or [ʰ] following the consonant. The symbol ['] following a stop indicates that it was not released. Notice the appropriate narrow transcription for the following words:

pay [pʰeɪ]	ape [eɪp']	pop [pʰɑp']
tea [tʰi]	eat [it']	tot [tʰɑt']
toe [tʰoʊ]	oat [oʊt']	tote [tʰoʊt']

Aspiration will also be altered when voiceless stops occur in consonant sequences, especially blends. For example, in prevocalic /s/ + stop blends ([sp], [st], and [sk]), coarticulation results in the stop being unaspirated. Strictly speaking, the appropriate symbol for stops in these conditions is [⁼] as opposed to the ['] used for unreleased stops. However, we will restrict our usage to the [ʰ] and ['] symbols to avoid confusion and "symbol overload." Consequently, we would narrowly transcribe the following words this way:

pie [pʰaɪ]	spy [sp'aɪ]
tow [tʰoʊ]	stow [st'oʊ]
key [kʰi]	ski [sk'i]

Although postvocalic singleton stops are usually unreleased, the same cannot be said for stops occurring in postvocalic nasal + stop blends such as -mp, -nt, and -nk. In these cases, each stop must be released with audible aspiration to distinguish it from the nasal consonant (in the same place of articulation) that precedes it. If a postvocalic blend is composed of two stops, the second stop must be released with audible aspiration to distinguish from the first. Notice the differences in audible aspiration in the following examples of narrow transcription:

lap [læp']	lamp [læmpʰ]	slip [slɪp']	slipped [slɪp't ʰ]
wet [wɛt']	went [wɛntʰ]	cook [kʰʊk']	cooked [kʰʊk'tʰ]
sick [sɪk']	sink [sɪŋkʰ]	rock [rɑk']	rocked [rɑk'tʰ]

Additional examples of the effect of aspiration will be found at the end of this chapter. Chapter 11 in the workbook includes additional rules and examples governing aspiration in mainstream American English.

ASSIMILATION PROCESSES

The effect of coarticulation may be rather minimal (as in the differences in /ʃ/ lip shaping for *she* and *shoe*), or it may actually cause changes in the identity of a phoneme, for example, in place, manner, or voicing. In these cases, the effect is referred to as **assimilation.**[1] Assimilation may be **progressive** or **regressive,**

---

[1]Phoneticians sometimes disagree over the concepts of coarticulation and assimilation. Some use the terms interchangeably, whereas others view coarticulation as the gestures that underlie pronunciation changes (Ohde & Sharf, 1992; Shriberg & Kent, 1982). These pronunciation changes, then, are seen as examples of assimilation. Ohde and Sharf (1992) point out that the disagreement is related to limited understanding of the nature of speech motor control. For our purposes, we will view assimilation as a product of coarticulation.

contiguous or **noncontiguous.** In progressive assimilation, an earlier occurring phoneme affects a phoneme that follows it in a word or phrase. The opposite is true of regressive assimilation. In this case, a later occurring phoneme alters the characteristic(s) of a phoneme preceding it. Assimilation is considered contiguous if the phonemes involved are immediately adjacent to each other. If one or more phonemes separate the phonemes involved in assimilation, it is considered noncontiguous. (See Table 6–1 for examples of assimilation.)

One way assimilation is seen is in contexts in which a phoneme takes on one or more of the characteristics of an adjacent phoneme but still retains its essential identity. For example, you learned that the liquids /l/ and /r/ are both produced with a voiced airstream. This is true, in the pure sense of their identities. However, if /r/ or /l/ is part of a consonant sequence with a voiceless consonant (e.g., *pray* or *clay*), it actually becomes **devoiced.** The essential identity of the palatal liquid or alveolar liquid is maintained despite the voicing alteration. The devoicing is a form of assimilation that occurs because of the overlapping articulatory movements involved when /r/ and /l/ are combined with voiceless consonants such as /p/, /k/, /f/, /θ/, /s/, and /ʃ/. (You can try this by putting your hand across your throat so that you can feel the laryngeal vibration. Say *lay,* then *play,* and note the difference in the timing of vibration for the /l/.) In these examples, assimilation is considered progressive because the earlier occurring phoneme (/p/, in this case) causes a change in the phoneme that follows it. It is also considered contiguous because the /p/ and liquid /l/ or /r/ are directly adjacent to each other.

An example of regressive assimilation can be found in the relationship between the nasal /n/ when it immediately precedes /k/ or /g/, as in *handkerchief.* Coarticulation results in the simplification of the [ndk] consonant sequence to [nk]. Then, the expected alveolar placement for [n] becomes velar, producing an [ŋ] because of the influence of the velar [k] that follows [ŋk]. The velar placement of a later sound ([k], [g]) can "back up" onto the place of an earlier sound ([n]). It is also an example of contiguous assimilation because the [n] and [k] are directly adjacent to each other.

We will take our example of noncontiguous assimilation from children's speech because this is when such effects are often likely to occur. One of the authors' children, as a toddler, sometimes produced the word *penny* as [pɛmi]. In this case, the alveolar [n] shifted to a bilabial nasal [m] because of progressive, noncontiguous assimilation (the effect of the bilabial [p]). Such assimilatory alterations are not unusual in the speech of very young children.

As you learn to transcribe phonemes in context and in connected speech, you will find that their sound properties can shift. This part of Chapter 6 demonstrates

TABLE 6–1   EXAMPLES OF ASSIMILATION: PLACE OF ARTICULATION

Example	Place Shift/Type
[bæθ sop] (bath soap)→[bæθ̪s̪op]	Dentalization; progressive, contiguous
[boʊθ sʌnz] (both suns)→[boʊθ̪s̪ʌnz]	Dentalization; progressive, contiguous
[hɔrs ʃu] (horseshoe)→[hɔr ʃːu]	Palatal; regressive, contiguous
[ples tʃenʤ] (place change)→[pleʃ tʃenʤ]	Palatal; regressive, contiguous
[kankwɛst] (conquest)→[kaŋkwɛst]	Velar; regressive, contiguous
[bænkwət] (banquet)→[bæŋkwət]	Velar; regressive, contiguous

such changes and how to record them. In some cases, you will transcribe a different phoneme than the one you might have expected. In other cases, you will learn to use **diacritic markings** to signal the alteration (but not complete change) of one or more phoneme characteristics. Diacritic markings allow you to specify the nature of an allophonic variation in your transcription. We will cover some, but not all, diacritic markings used in the IPA. We have selected those that we have found particularly useful in applying phonetics to our everyday work. In this chapter, our examples will be drawn from normal adult speech. Later, in Chapter 9, we will return to this topic with examples from the speech of children with normal and disordered speech.

PLACE OF ARTICULATION

There are a number of alterations in place of articulation that may occur as a result of assimilation. Some result in a complete change; others, in a slight shift of place. Typical examples follow.

DENTALIZATION   You have learned that there are two interdental phonemes: /θ/ and /ð/. If /θ/ or /ð/ is adjacent to an alveolar phoneme (/t/, /d/, /s/, /z/, /n/, or /l/), the alveolar phoneme may shift to a dental place of articulation. Try this for yourself by saying these two phrases and noting your tongue placement for /s/: *less time, less thought*. Notice that your tongue tip remains on your alveolar ridge for the first phrase because the alveolar [s] is followed by another alveolar consonant, [t]. When [s] is followed by [θ], however, the position for [s] shifts so that it is more against the teeth. The diacritic marking for **dentalization** is [͜], and *less thought* would be narrowly transcribed as [lɛs̪θɔt].

OTHER CHANGES IN PLACE OF ARTICULATION   You have already read about one of these examples of place change: the shift of [n] to the velar [ŋ] when it directly precedes a velar [k] or [g] (as in *handkerchief*). There are many other examples of assimilation in English involving other places of articulation. One everyday example can be found in the pronunciation of *grandma* and *grandpa* as [græmə] and [græmpə]. Notice that it is much easier to say the transcribed words than to try to pronounce every phoneme in *grandma* and *grandpa*. The demands of rapid speech require economy of movement. In this case, the [d] is omitted (see the section on Elision/ Omission/Haplology), and the alveolar [n] becomes a bilabial [m], just like the place of the phonemes that follow it ([m] and [p]). (See Table 6–1 for additional examples of assimilation involving place of articulation.) For practice in narrow transcription of place changes, refer to the exercises at the end of this chapter and to Chapter 13 in the workbook.

VOICING EFFECTS

We noted earlier in this chapter that voicing can also be affected by assimilation. Not only can a voiced phoneme become partially voiceless, but a voiceless phoneme can become partially voiced, depending on phonetic context. We will begin with the first type, devoicing of a consonant.

As we noted earlier, /r/ and /l/ are considered voiced consonants. However, when blended with a preceding voiceless consonant (forming a consonant sequence), /r/ and /l/ are produced almost without voicing. [r] and [l] have no voiceless cognate. Consequently, the appropriate diacritic marking to use for this partial loss of voicing from a normally voiced consonant is [̥]. The marking looks like a very small, open circle, placed directly under the phoneme affected. Thus, appropriate narrow transcription of *tree* would be [t r̥ i]. Similarly, *slot* would be narrowly transcribed as [s l̥ ɑ t]. You might try saying the following word pairs and noticing that [r] and [l] are definitely voiced in the first word and have almost no voicing in the second of each pair:

ray [reɪ]—pray [pr̥eɪ]	lie [laɪ]—ply [pl̥aɪ]
rue [ru]—true [tr̥u]	lay [leɪ]—play [pl̥eɪ]
rye [raɪ]—fry [fr̥aɪ]	low [loʊ]—slow [sl̥oʊ]
row [roʊ]—crow [kr̥oʊ]	Lee [li]—flee [fl̥i]

Another voicing effect appears as **intervocalic voicing.** In this case, a voiceless phoneme is surrounded by voiced phonemes, for example, the [t] in *butter.* As a result, the allophone of /t/ in this word may be heard with a range of voicing. It could be produced as an audibly aspirated stop [tʰ], as in [bʌtʰ ɚ]. Or [t] might become totally voiced, soundling like [bʌdɚ]. It is quite likely, however, that a partially voiced [t] will result because of the voiced sounds around it [bʌ t̬ ɚ]. The diacritic marking to indicate partial voicing looks like a lowercase, orthographic *v*, and it is placed under the affected phoneme. Another consonant frequently affected by intervocalic voicing is /h/ in words such as *birdhouse* and *behind* (transcribed as [b ɝ d h̬ aʊ s] and [bi h̬ aɪ nd], respectively. Because /h/ has no voiced cognate, we use the [̬] symbol to indicate the partial voicing that occurs as a consequence of coarticulation. For practice in narrow transcription of voicing changes, see the exercises at the end of this chapter and in Chapter 14 of the workbook.

RESONANCE / NASALITY

Vowels may be affected by another assimilatory effect associated with nasal consonants. Often in connected speech, a vowel sound adjacent to a nasal consonant takes on nasal resonance. This is usually the case for a vowel preceded and followed by a nasal consonant, as in the word *moon.* Try saying these two words and listening for a difference in vowel resonance: *boot* ([b u t]), *moon* [m u n]. Even though the vowel is the same (/u/) in each word, it is more "nasal sounding" in *moon.* Because the vowel assumes some nasal resonant quality, we use a diacritic marking to indicate this effect, [~]. Thus, narrow transcription of *moon* would be [m ũ n]. Assimilation nasality may also affect vowels immediately preceding a nasal consonant. For practice in narrow transcription of **nasal assimilation,** see the exercises at the end of this chapter and also Chapter 13 in the workbook.

OTHER PHONOLOGICAL PROCESSES

ELISION / OMISSION / HAPLOLOGY

A number of speech sounds and even syllables may be omitted in connected speech as a result of coarticulation. The /h/ and /ð/ are two consonants especially prone to this effect. They are frequently dropped in rapid connected speech, as in *Where is he?* ([w ɛ r ɪ z i]) and *Stop them!* ([s t ɑ p ə m].[2] Final consonants of words occasionally may be omitted during rapid speech, such as *Let me go!* ([l ɛ m i g oʊ]. When just one consonant or a few consecutive consonants are omitted in this way, the term applied is **elision.**

Words such as *sixths* and *guests* also provide us with examples of elision occurring in response to the demands of rapid connected speech. With consonant sequences such as *-sts,* two sounds that are essentially the same are separated by an intervening sound. The demands of rapid speech often result in the loss of the intervening consonants along with elongation of the first sound. For example, *sixths* ([s ɪ k s̩ θ s̩]) may be produced as [s ɪ k s:] (remember that the symbol [:] indicates increased duration). Similarly, *desks* ([d ɛ s k s]) is more easily produced as [d ɛ s:]. Production of *asks* ([æ s k s]) as [æ s:] is another example of this type of omission, as is the production of *mirror* [m ɪ r ɚ] as [m ɪ r :].

In some cases in connected speech, whole syllables may be omitted. **Haplology** is the term used to describe what can happen when two very similar syllables occur in close succession. *Mississippi* (four syllables) is often pronounced as [m ɪs ɪp i] (three syllables) by natives of the state. Similarly, *Coca-Cola* (four syllables) may be heard as [koʊkoʊlə]. Generally, listeners will understand these changes without difficulty. Further examples of omissions due to coarticulation may be found at the end of this chapter and in Chapter 15 in the workbook.

ADDITION / EPENTHESIS

At the beginning of this chapter, we gave you an example of a consonant addition (intrusive /w/) in the expressions *so easy* ([s o w i z i]) and *to each* ([t u w i ʧ]). In connected speech, the [w] and [j] are sometimes intruded in order to separate vowels that end one word and begin another. The type of intruded consonant depends on the height and position of the first vowel. In the following examples, notice that [w] follows high back vowels and [j] follows high front vowels:

New England	[n u w ɪ ŋ g l ə n d]	see Ann	[s i j æ n]
so old	[s o w oʊ l d]	my apple	[m aɪ j æ p l̩]
bow out	[b aʊ w aʊ t]	stay in	[s t eɪ j ɪ n]

Instead of a [w] or a [j], a **glottal stop** may intrude in these same types of coarticulatory environments. The glottal stop is produced at the glottis by rapidly closing the vocal folds tightly, then releasing them to continue voicing. It is especially needed to separate *the* from a following vowel-initiated word. For example, *the apple* needs an intrusive [ʔ] or [j] to be most easily understood: [ð i j æ p l̩] or [ð i ʔ æ p l̩]. In phrases such as *he eats* ([h i ʔ i t s] or [h i j i t s], an intrusive [ʔ] or [j] is important to distinguish the phrase from the word *heats* [h i: t s], which is produced with an elongated vowel. Notice how a glottal stop or a glide may intrude in the following examples:

---

[2]It is even more probable that the [ə] will also be deleted and the /m/ will become a syllabic [m], as discussed in the section Duration in this chapter.

we even	[w i ʔ i v n̩]	[w i j i v n̩]
the only	[ð i ʔ oʊn l i]	[ð i j oʊ n l i]
two apples	[t u ʔ æ p ḷ z]	[t u w æ p ḷ z]

The glottal stop or [j] can also occur in [l] + [ɪn] combinations in words such as *seeing* (e.g., [s i ʔ ɪ ŋ] or [s i j ɪ ŋ]. Further examples of coarticulation involving [w], [j], and [ʔ] may be found at the end of this chapter and in Chapter 15 of the workbook.

Another manner of articulation, an intrusive stop, is likely to occur if a nasal resonant consonant immediately precedes a voiceless fricative such as /s/ or /θ/. The stop will be voiceless, with closure in the same place of articulation as the nasal consonant. Thus, in a word like *warmth*, a [p] will intrude: [w ɔ r m p θ]. In a word such as *chance*, an alveolar [t] intrudes: [ʧ æ n t s]. Finally, the word *strength* gives us an example of [k] intrusion due to coarticulation: [s t r ɛ ŋ k θ]. More examples can be found at the end of this chapter and in Chapter 15 of the workbook.

SUMMARY: INFLUENCE OF CONTEXT

By now you are aware of how phonemes can vary in production in connected speech. Phonemes may be omitted, added, or completely or partially change their identity, depending on the demands of connected speech. We noted earlier that these adjustments make speech production more efficient. They also have another effect: they make a speaker sound more "natural" or "native." Some speakers of English as a second language tend to produce speech as if they were reading words, slowly and deliberately. This decreases coarticulatory effects and makes the speaker sound more "foreign." In the second part of the chapter, we will discuss another important part of the "naturalness" of speaking a language: suprasegmentals.

SPEECH RHYTHM AND SUPRASEGMENTAL FEATURES

If you listen to speakers of languages other than English, for example, French, Hindi, or Swedish, you will probably first note that you cannot understand what they are saying. If you keep listening to these speakers, you may notice that some of their phonemes (also known as **segments** of speech) do not sound like anything you have ever heard in English, either. What you will also notice is that, regardless of the phonemes and words, the language does not necessarily "sound" like English. French has more of a "flow" or a different "sound" than English. For that matter, British English does not "sound" like mainstream American English. An important part of the sound of different languages is the result of the **suprasegmental aspects** of speech. Other terms that have been applied to this phenomenon include speech melody and prosody. Suprasegmental aspects of speech are most simply defined as features of speech over and above phoneme segments, especially aspects of speech rhythm. They include accent, emphasis, phrasing, and timing.

THE SYLLABLE: BASIC UNIT OF SPEECH RHYTHM

The basic unit of speech rhythm is the **syllable.** Although this sounds simple, the concept of what constitutes a syllable has been a source of intense study and scientific argument over the years. Most recently, Shriberg and Kent (1995) advanced the sonority theory to explain the definition of a syllable. **Sonority** refers to the relative loudness of speech sounds. Some phonemes, especially vowels, have greater sonority than other phonemes because they are produced with more energy. A phoneme's sonority is determined in relation to the relative loudness of other phonemes that share similar length, pitch, and stress. For each spoken syllable, there is a **sonorant peak,** or a speech segment of maximum energy. That sonorant peak is most often identified as a vowel. Consonants that may or may not surround a vowel form a **trough,** with less energy. If a syllable consists of a vowel only (e.g., *oh* and *eye*), only a sonorant peak is identified. If more than one sonorant peak is heard, then more than one syllable is heard. Thus, current thought views a syllable as always being characterized by a sonorant peak (usually a vowel). This sonorant peak, then, is the basic unit of speech rhythm.

A syllable may consist only of a vowel or may be composed of a vowel and adjacent consonant(s). Consonants can begin or end a syllable, but they do not function as the essential part, or sonorant peak. The only exception is syllabic consonants, mentioned earlier in this chapter. Syllables that end in a vowel are termed **open** (e.g., *tea* and *my*), whereas those that end in a consonant are **closed** (e.g., *mat* and *sit*). The most common syllable shape in English is the CV (consonant + vowel). Examples would be the *re-* in *refill* and the *pa-* in *paper*. Another commonly occurring syllable shape is the CVC, such as the *-ton* in *Washington,* and the *-sic* in *music*. The VC syllable shape (e.g., *on-* in the word *onset*) occurs less often. The "largest" syllable that is found in English is CCCVCCCC. An example of this syllable shape is found in the word *strengths* ([s t r ɛ ŋ k θ s]. However, a syllable cannot contain more than one vowel or sonorant peak. If it does, it will be perceived as more than one syllable. For example, the word *seeing* contains a CV ([s i]) and a VC ([ɪŋ]). *Seeing* would sound very similar to *sing* if it were not for the unisyllable-bisyllable distinction.

Syllable composition or shape influences coarticulation and relates to the timing of speech. The average American English syllable duration is .02 seconds. Of course, this is just an average. There will be some variations of syllable duration according to individual speaker differences and stress patterns. If you pronounce two similar syllables with equal stress, they will have roughly the same duration. For example, try saying the words *catch* and *scratch* with the same amount of stress. With equal stress, they will have pretty much the same duration. Remember our example of alterations in vowel duration according to the following consonant, earlier in this chapter? The words *buy* and *bite,* when spoken with equal stress, will be very similar in duration. The [aɪ], which has a longer duration in *buy,* is shortened by the intrinsic coarticulation required in a syllable in the CVC word *bite*. Rather than hearing phonemes presented individually and irregularly, you hear them coarticulated in syllable units. These units help you recognize each phoneme because of the transitional characteristics of consonant-vowel and vowel-consonant **junctures.** These junctures supply you with important perceptual information. Furthermore, coarticulation effects extend beyond the syllable, as noted earlier in this chapter.

In this part of the chapter, we will focus on American English **accent, emphasis, phrasing, intonation,** and **rate.** These nonlinguistic aspects of speech result from the interaction of variations in loudness, pitch, and duration of syllables as they occur in connected phrases and pauses. The result is a speech signal with additional information that influences meaning, assists in listening and understanding, and makes speech more interesting.

ACCENT

Accent is one form of speech stress. **Stress** points out, sets apart, focuses on, or otherwise gives vocal prominence to a unit of speech. Accent, in particular, refers to the stress given to a syllable within a word in comparison with that word's other syllables. (Stress can also vary across words in a phrase or sentence, as you will discover later in this chapter.) English is referred to as a stress-timed language because in every word of more than one syllable, a syllable will be stressed above the others. Additionally, stressed syllables are audibly different from those of lesser stress. Other languages that have a more regular beat and do not observe variable stressing are called syllable-timed. Even within English dialects, the difference between heavily stressed and unstressed syllables can vary. American English uses less difference between heavily stressed and unstressed syllables than British English. As a result, syllables that are pronounced in American English may be omitted in British English. For example, the word *secretary* is produced with four syllables [ˈs ɛ k r ə t ɛ r i] but with only three syllables [ˈs ɛ k r ə t r i] by British English speakers. (See Chapter 8 for more information.)

We will cover the three basic levels of accent in American English: primary, secondary, and unaccented syllables. The sonorant peak, or vowel, is the syllable element that actually changes with accent, not the consonants. An accented syllable will be made with greater physiological force, which produces a syllable with (1) greater loudness, (2) greater duration, and (3) a rise in pitch. An unaccented syllable will have reduced force in production, resulting in reduced loudness and duration as well as a lowered pitch. Many speakers use a combination of both stressing and destressing syllables to produce accenting in their connected speech. Thus, the contrast or ratio between accented and unaccented syllables can be made by expanding (accenting) a stressed syllable, reducing force of production (deaccented syllable), or a combination of both. Different speakers can vary in their use of accent levels, depending on the utterance. Also, accenting can vary according to dialectic variation. (Consider the accent difference between these mainstream American English and Appalachian English productions of *theater*: [ˈθ i j ə t ɚ] (primary accent on first syllable), as opposed to [θ i ˈj eɪ t ɚ] (primary accent on the second syllable). Despite these individual variations, we can still discuss general rules for assigning accent levels and also provide exercises to help you develop this skill. Understanding of accent is crucial to effective communication. It also is important in programming for individuals with speech disorders, particularly children with intelligibility problems (see Chapter 9 for further details on this topic).

Given our emphasis on the IPA in this book, we will use IPA graphic depiction symbols to mark accent differences. You mark a syllable with a primary accent by placing a vertical mark [ˈ] above and to the left of it, for example, *simple* is transcribed as [ˈs i m p l̩]. For secondary accent, you place the same vertical mark [ˌ] below and to the left of the affected syllable. Unaccented syllables are unmarked. Thus, narrow transcription of the word *peppercorn* would be [ˈp ɛ p ɚ ˌk ɔ r n]. The counterparts of these marks in a dictionary would be a heavy accent mark (´) following the syllable with primary accent and a lighter accent mark (´) following a syllable with secondary accent. Depending on your reasons for taking a phonetics course, you or your instructor may find one set of markings preferable or more useful than the other. However, we will continue using the "official" IPA symbols throughout this textbook and in your workbook.

Rules for assigning stress in English can seem very erratic because deciding which syllable to accent is largely a matter of following conventional usage. There are some general rules that can be observed in assigning syllable stress. We will begin with bisyllabic words and examples. In bisyllabic words, there is a strong tendency for the first syllable to receive the primary accent, for example, *making* ['m eɪ kɪŋ], and *mainly* ['m eɪ n l i]. This rule holds especially true when the accented syllable precedes suffixes such as *-ing, -er, -est, -cious,* and *-tion.* In contrast, the accented syllable usually follows unaccented prefixes such as *a-, be-, re-, de-, ad-,* and *ex-.* See Table 6–2 for examples of stress assignment for different bisyllabic words.

It may help you to understand how to listen for accenting and to realize how important conventional usage is by trying the following exercise. Because you expect to hear normal stressing patterns, you may not understand familiar words when the accent is transposed. Try to pronounce the following words with the primary accent as indicated, and see how unfamiliar they may sound.

Ameri´ca	ener´getic	dependent´
sylla´ble	emotion´al	intensi´ty
inter´esting	inton´ation	cate´gorize
foundation´	secretar´y	con´sider

Do these words suddenly sound unfamiliar? One reason for the differences is that pronunciation changes almost automatically as we change accenting. Unstressed syllables tend to have /ə/ for their nucleus; the full vowel identity is neutralized by the lack of stress. For example, notice how the pronunciation of *-i-* [ɪ] in *America* can change, depending on the syllable accented: *Amer´ica* [ə 'm ɛ r ə k ə] (shift from [ɪ] to [ə]) but *Ameri´ca* [ə m ə' r ɪ k ə] (shift from [ə] to [ɪ]). Likewise, in the word *syllable,* the *-a-* changes from [ə] to [eɪ] or [ɑ] when it is given unconventional stress: ['s ɪ l ə b l̩] to [sə 'l æ b l̩] or [s ə 'l ɑ b l̩].

Accented syllables are likely to follow their usual vowel spelling pronunciation, as described in Chapter 3. However, the vowels in unaccented syllables often change. The diphthongs /eɪ/ and /o ʊ/ become pure vowels /e/ and /o/ when unstressed, except when they occur in final, open syllables. Thus, transcription of *-o-* in *location* would be [l o 'k eɪ ʃ ə n], but *window* would be transcribed [w ɪ n d o ʊ]. (See Chapter 16 in the workbook for practice in transcribing these changes.) For the vowels /i/, /æ/, /u/, and /ɑ/, loss of primary stress leads to their pronuncia-

TABLE 6–2 EXAMPLES OF STRESS ASSIGNMENT FOR DIFFERENT BISYLLABIC WORDS

cupcake	['kʌpkek]	happy	['hæpi]	above	[ə'bʌv]
saddle	['sædl̩]	biggest	['bɪgəst]	reply	[ri'plaɪ]
market	['mɑrkət]	sunny	['sʌni]	detain	[di'teɪn]
taco	['tɑkoʊ]	faded	['feɪdəd]	admire	[æd'maɪr]
column	['kɑləm]	station	['steɪʃən]	extent	[ɛks'tɛnt]

TABLE 6–3 WORD PAIRS FOR PHONEMIC STRESS

per´fect	adjective: [p ɜ˞ f ɪ k t]	→	perfect´	verb: [p ɚ f ɛ k t]
pro´gress	noun: [p r ɑ g r ɛ s]	→	progress´	verb: [p r o ˈg r ɛ s]
re´bel	noun: [ˈr ɛ b l̩]	→	rebel´	verb: [r ɪ ˈb ɛ l]
con´flict	noun: [ˈk ɑ n f l ɪ k t]	→	conflict´	verb: [k ə n ˈf l ɪ k t]
ab´stract	adjective: [ˈæ b s t r æ k t]	→	abstract´	verb: [æ b ˈs t r æ k t]
com´plex	noun: [ˈk ɑ m p l ɛ k s]	→	complex´	adjective: [k ə m ˈp l ɛ k s]

tion as /ɪ/, /ɛ/, /ʊ/, and /ʌ/, respectively. Further deaccenting will reduce these vowels to /ə/. Thus, you might hear *relief* as [r i ˈl i f], [r̩ ɪ ˈl i f], or [r ə ˈl i f], depending on the degree of deaccenting of the first syllable.

Accent can also be **phonemic;** that is, a change in syllable accent changes syllable pronunciation and, consequently, word meaning. Table 6–3 gives examples of phonemic stress.

Other examples of phonemic accenting occur in the following words when primary accent shifts from the first to the last syllable: *survey, suspect, torment, transport, subject, reject, produce, digest, escort, insult, exile, content,* and *recess.*

At other times syllable accent may change without altering meaning. Such pronunciation differences often reflect dialect variations. In mainstream American English, for example, you may say *adult* as a ´dult *or* adult´ without altering meaning. Compare your pronunciation of these words with those of a friend or acquaintance: *automobile, cigarette, concrete, contrary, defense, dictator, gasoline, illustrate,* and *locate.* For these words, accent may be different, but it is not a phonemic change.

Word meaning can also change depending on the presence or absence of secondary accent. This is especially noticeable in words that take the suffix *-ate.* Table 6–4 shows the shift in pronunciation ([ə] to [e]) that occurs when *-ate* is added.

Usually, secondary accent is also present in compound words; these are formed from two other words. In such words, the second syllable is almost never reduced to /ə/. Examples include *air´plane* [ˈɛ r p l e n], *hot´dog* [ˈhɑt ˌdɔ g], *cow´boy* [ˈk aʊ ˌb ɔ ɪ], and *base´ball* [ˈb eɪ s ˌb ɔ l].

For unaccented syllables, destressing may even lead to loss of /ə/, particularly when a following resonant consonant is **homorganic** (made in the same position with the same articulator) with the previous consonant. Because [t] and [l] are both lingua-alveolars in the word *cattle,* pronunciation may be either [ˈk æ t ə l] or [ˈk æ t l̩]. In this case (and others like it), the stress is so reduced that the syllabic [l] can take on the function of a syllable nucleus. Other familiar examples of this phenomenon are found in *kitten* [ˈk ɪ t n̩], *button* [ˈbʌ t n̩], and *little* [ˈl ɪ t l̩].

TABLE 6–4 PRONUNCIATION SHIFTS RESULTING FROM THE PRESENCE OF SECONDARY ACCENT

No Secondary Accent		Secondary Accent Present	
deli´berate	adjective: [d ɪ ˈl ɪ b r ə t]	deli´berate´	verb: [d ə ˈlɪ bɚ ˌe t]
affil´iate	noun: [ə ˈf ɪ l i j ə t]	affil´iate´	verb: [ə ˈf ɪ l i j e t]
del´egate	noun: [ˈd ɛ l ə g ə t]	del´egate´	verb: [dɛ l ə ˌg e t]
gra´duate	noun: [ˈg r æ ʤu ə t]	gra´duate´	verb: [g r æ ʤ u ˌe t]

In the most extreme form of stress reduction, an unstressed syllable will be completely omitted. This occurs quite often in British English, as noted earlier in this chapter. There are also a number of words that may lose syllables in mainstream American English:

	Formal	Conversational
annual	[ˈæ n j u ə l]	[ˈæ n j ʊ l]
evening	[ˈi v ə n ɪ ŋ]	[ˈi v n ɪ ŋ]
family	[ˈf æ m ə l i]	[ˈf æ m l i]
miniature	[ˈm ɪ n i ə tʃ ɚ]	[ˈm ɪ n j ə tʃ ɚ]

You can find numerous examples in the workbook to help you to recognize the different levels of accent (see especially Chapter 16). You will begin by simply counting the number of syllables, then move on to marking the primary accent. In later workbook exercises, you will learn to mark the secondary accent and identify the /ə/ characteristic of unstressed syllables. If you have difficulty determining the stressed syllable in a word, try saying the word with stress on a different syllable each time. For example, try saying *ob´stacle, obsta´cle, obstacle´*. Which one "sounds" correct? Right, the first pronunciation, with primary stress on the first syllable: [ˈɑ b s t ə k ə l]. (Feeling discouraged? Remember, you have come a long way in learning the IPA since you started with the vowels; marking for accent is just another step along the way.)

EMPHASIS

Emphasis affects units larger than the syllable. In particular, it refers to the stressing of a word or words within a phrase or sentence. Like accent, emphasis is produced primarily by greater physiologic force. This results in increased loudness and duration of syllables within the stressed word(s), along with an accompanying pitch change. Conversely, some other words may be deemphasized because of reduced force. You may also achieve emphasis by using pauses between words or by elongating the duration of a particular syllable. Like levels of accent, levels of emphasis are variable and difficult to specify—but even more so. Emphasis may be marked in different ways, including use of <u>underlining</u> and <u>double underlining</u> or *italics* and **bold type.**

Unlike accent, the application of emphasis does not follow either consistently recurring patterns or conventional usage. How you apply stress in your speech is personal and relates to your communicative intent. If your communicative intent changes, you will change your stress as a result. Emphasis adds information to an utterance over and above the phoneme segments, their grouping into syllables, and their syllable accent pattern. If you want to draw attention to a particular word label, then you emphasize the label accordingly: "The <u>last</u> house is on the <u>right</u>." If you are trying to reiterate or stress a point, you might use emphasis this way: "I said I <u>don't</u> want to go." Perhaps you are contrasting parallel thoughts: "<u>I</u> can be here at <u>six</u>, but <u>she</u> can't come until <u>seven</u>." Notice how the meaning of a sentence can change, depending on the emphasis:

<u>I</u> need some sleep!   (Emphasis on who needs sleep; you may not, but I do.)

I <u>need</u> some sleep!   (I don't just want it; I need it.)

I need <u>some</u> sleep!   (Emphasis on minimum amount needed; without rest, I can't function.)

I need some <u>sleep</u>!   (I've had enough to eat/drink; now I need to rest.)

Sometimes emphasis is used to distinguish a compound word from an adjective + noun combination. For example, a baby may sit in a <u>high</u>chair [h aɪ tʃ ɛ r], but you may choose to sit in a high<u>chair</u> [h aɪ 'tʃ ɛ r] at the breakfast counter in a restaurant. You might specifically see a red-winged <u>black</u>bird ['b l æ k b ɚ d] in the spring, or you might see just some unidentifiable black <u>bird</u> [b l æ k 'b ɚ d]. Word pairs such as <u>green</u>house ['g r i n h aʊ s] (where plants are grown) and *green house* [g r i n 'h aʊ s] (the house painted green) also follow this pattern. Another example is <u>hot</u> dog [h ɑ t ˌd ɔ g] (something to eat) and hot dog [h ɑ t ˈd ɔ g] (a panting poodle).

Deemphasis of a word is also possible. When it occurs, it is similar to the reduction of unaccented syllables. Frequently used, short, connective words such as *was, of, the,* and *a* are almost never emphasized. Instead, they are usually produced as /ə/ in connected speech. Thus, "Do you have to go?" would most likely be transcribed as [ˈd u j ə ˈh æ f t ə ˈgoʊ]. This deemphasis explains why expressions such as *want to, have to,* and *got to* are most often pronounced as *wanta, hafta,* and *gotta* in the connected speech of both adults and children.

PHRASING

A **speech phrase** consists of a continuous utterance, bounded by silent intervals. Intervals between phrases are called **pauses.** Your speech phrasing is related to your breathing but does not necessarily reflect your actual breathing pattern. When you inhale for speech in conversation, you do it in a pause between phrases. You do not have to inhale for each phrase, however. More than one phrase can be said on a single breath, for example, "She saw the guests arrive, and then she went downstairs." In this example, you may pause between *arrive* and *and,* but you should be able to complete the sentence (and a few more) on one breath.

In writing, phrases can be marked by punctuation marks such as commas, periods, semicolons, colons, question marks, and exclamation marks. These written punctuation conventions do not necessarily correspond to your speech phrasing, though. For example, the written expression "red, white, and blue" has commas to separate elements. More than likely, however, you would say a continuous phrase in speech: [r ɛ d w aɪ t n̩ b l u] rather than pausing between each color name. On the other hand, you might insert pauses when punctuation would not signal their presence, for example, "Today [pause] is the last day [pause] of class!"

Several methods have been suggested for marking phrases. You can use either method with orthographic symbols or with IPA symbols. One suggested method is the use of a **ligature,** or curved underlining. Thus, for our sentence in the last paragraph, we could mark phrasing this way: "Today is the last day of class." Another way to indicate pauses can be to insert one, two, or three lines between words, depending on the length of the pause (shorter to longer). Again, with the previous sentence, we could mark the phrasing this way:

Today /// is the last day // of class!

[tuˈdeɪ] /// [ɪzðəˈlæstdeɪ] // [əvˈklæs]

You will notice that the phonetic symbols within a phrase are transcribed consecutively, without interruption for word boundaries. This indicates junctures that are coarticulated. You may use spaces, therefore, to mark phrase boundaries and eliminate the lines to mark pauses (unless you want to indicate relative duration of the pauses). In other words, there is more than one way to indicate phrasing in connected speech. Your choice of system will probably depend on your purpose(s) for transcribing as well as your instructor's preference. Marking for phrasing is much more frequently used for public speaking scripts than for error transcription in speech-language pathology, for instance.

The speaker determines which and how many words to link together in a phrase, as well as the duration of pauses. These decisions affect the listener's ability to understand the message. Reasons for using phrasing patterns include

1. To group the words of a thought into a unit
2. To create emphasis
3. For parenthetical comments
4. To accommodate difficult listening situations

The use of phrasing to present units of meaning is particularly important for listener understanding. "We went to the store / because we were hungry" makes sense. But "We went to the / store because we / were hungry" interferes with, rather than facilitates, understanding. Similarly, pauses can be used for emphasis: "I want to go // now // not later." (Translation: Let's get moving!) In addition, the word *now* will probably be uttered with longer duration and a higher pitch. Parenthetical remarks are conversational asides, for example, "The weather // I hope // is going to get better." In this case, "I hope" will probably have lower loudness and pitch than the rest of the utterance.

A sensitive speaker also takes listeners and listening conditions into account. If you were speaking in a noisy room to someone with a hearing loss, you would probably use shorter phrases and more pauses to aid the person's understanding. In class, your instructor uses shorter phrases and longer pauses when presenting new, unfamiliar, or especially difficult material. Listener age, ability to listen, and speaking environment can all influence the use of phrasing.

You also use pauses to formulate your next phrase or phrases when you are speaking extemporaneously. If you are speaking rapidly in conversation, you may need to pause to gather your thoughts. Sometimes such pauses are marked with fillers such as "um," "uh," "well," and "I guess." These pauses give you time to think and formulate exactly what you wish to say as well as to add emphasis and meaning.

Overall, phrasing is another aspect of speaking that you must control as a speaker. Your message is not just composed of words made up of phonemes. Effective communication also requires use of accent, emphasis, phrasing patterns, and intonation (covered in the next section of this chapter).

INTONATION

You have learned that accent reflects changes in syllables within a word, whereas emphasis reflects changes in the words in a phrase. Intonation, however, involves changes over an entire phrase. What changes in intonation is the rising and falling of pitch. In English, these pitch inflections result in audible **intonation contours,** which can add meaning over and above the phonemes, accent pattern, and emphasis pattern used. Thus, the contours typically enhance, but do not change, meaning in English. However, in tonal languages, such as Chinese and Japanese, syllable pitch changes actually can indicate differences in meaning. That is, the same CVC syllable [g aɪ] can have different meanings, depending on the pitch level or pitch change at which it is said. We will focus here on the intonation characteristics typical of English, however.

The description of intonation contours requires describing (1) the degree of pitch change, (2) the direction of change, and (3) the rate of change. Because your fundamental voice pitch varies as you speak (centering on an average), intonation is marked by pitch changes that are relatively different from each other, not from an absolute, unchanging pitch. Four relative pitch levels are conventionally recognized in American English intonation. Level 2 is a standard or baseline for a phrase, from which the speaker drops to 1 or rises to 3. Level 4 is reserved for expressions of surprise or high emotional excitement. You can depict intonation by using the respective numbers for each word or syllable, as shown below:

3   3

Hurry up!   He's coming!

2   2

Direction and rate of pitch change can also be depicted by using straight and slanting lines to mark the levels. The examples below illustrate use of this marking system.

Hurry up! He's coming!

My goodness!

Remember that these markings, although sufficient for indicating intonation, will correlate only roughly with measured variations in fundamental voice frequency. Nevertheless, they can be particularly useful when such a system is needed.

Many intonation patterns result, in part, from pitch changes caused by application of accent and emphasis. The following sentence illustrates this:

I lost my calculator.

The word *calculator* is a key word to be emphasized above the rest of the sentence by greater intensity and duration and by a rise in fundamental voice frequency. Normally, the accent pattern of *calculator* would be [k æ l k j ə ˌle t ɚ]. Because the word occurs at the end of the utterance, the unstressed syllables will be even more heavily deaccented than usual. Not only will *calculator* be lower in intensity and shorter in duration, it will have an audible pitch drop, below the rest of the phrase. Emphasis, in order to aid meaning, determines that intonation will change primarily on *calculator,* the emphasized word. These parts of the intonation contour are dictated by accent and emphasis. The unusual drop in pitch on the final syllables, however, is the result of intonation that tells the listener something new. "Here," it says, "the utterance is now completed." Compare the intonation contours in these sentences:

I lost my calculator.

I lost my calculator, my pen, and my pencil.

In the second sentence, the rising intonation on *calculator,* with the help of appropriate phrasing, tells the listener "Keep listening; there's more to come." Consider the sentence "We bought *knives, forks, dishes,* and *spoons.*" Use of rising pitch on *knives, forks,* and *dishes* signals your listener that there is more to come in the series. Conversely, the dropping pitch for *spoons* indicates the completion of the series and the utterance. In this example, the end of the series is also marked by the word *and,* occurring just before the last word. Consequently, both *and* and the intonation contour provide complementary and redundant information to aid the listener. Try to say this sentence again without *and* but with appropriate intonation. Now, try it again, including *and* but using the same intonation rise on *knives, forks, dishes,* and *spoons.* Which of the sentences is easiest to understand: (1) the one without *and,* (2) the one containing *and* but accompanied by consistent intonation across all items, or (3) the one with both *and* and the varied intonation contour? Notice how the sentence is most easily understood when it includes *and* with the varied intonation contour.

You have now learned two uses of intonation: to indicate a series and to indicate termination of an utterance. Another important use of intonation is in signaling a question. Consider the statement "They will." If said with a slight drop in intonation, you hear it as a statement. But, if you say it with rising intonation, it becomes a question. Because we do not have question marks in speaking, as we do in writing, we mark the difference by intonation contour.

In "They will?" the intonation contour influences the meaning very strongly. Another example of intonation contour actually altering meaning can be found in the expression *oh* [oʊ]. The syllable does not have a meaning of its own but can actually convey meaning through intonation. The following common intonation messages demonstrate this point:

Carrier	Intonation Message
oh	I'm still listening to you.
oh\	I understand.
oh\	Now I finally understand it.
oh/	Really, are you sure?
ohoh	Now you're in trouble.

You may use intonation carriers in conversation, especially to signal your conversation partner that you are listening but that you do not want to interrupt him or her. Carriers such as *uhuh* [ʌ h ʌ], *mmm* [m:], and *yes* [j ɛs] are commonly used. Use of *mmhum* [m: hm:] even allows you to keep your mouth closed while still indicating that you are paying attention. Notice how intonation contours carry meaning in the following:

Carrier	Information
uh huh	I'm still listening.
uh/huh	I understand.

Carrier	Information
uh/huh	I didn't know that or That's really interesting.
mmmmmm	I'm still listening.
mmmmmm	Is that so?
mmmmmm	I didn't know that or That's really interesting.

Even the standard "Hello" can convey a meaning with intonation:

Carrier	Information
hello	I am pleased to meet you.
hello	I am very pleased to meet you.
hello	What do you want with me? (telephone greeting)

We can identify a great variety of intonation contours. They are influenced by a speaker's accent and intonation patterns, length of the phrase, linguistic intent of the message, and emotional affect. Three recurring intonation contours that might be considered conventional usage of mainstream American English can be identified: falling intonation, rising intonation, and rising-falling intonation.

FALLING INTONATION   This pattern signals the end of completion of an utterance and suggests to the listener that no verbal response is necessary. It occurs most often at the end of a phrase, accompanied by decreased intensity and syllable duration and vowels reduced to /ə/. Examples of this falling intonation occur in phrases such as "That's all" and "It's over."

RISING INTONATION   This contour indicates that a response is expected of the listener or that the speaker is not finished with the message. It marks items in a series, such as "the knife, fork, dishes, and spoon." It can also indicate a question that most likely requires a yes-no answer, for example, "Are you coming home?" or "Is that all?"

RISING-FALLING INTONATION   A common intonation contour, this one is used in making a simple statement of fact or giving a command. Examples include "The store is closed now" and "Come here." *Wh* questions (initiated by *where, when, why,* and *what*) also often follow this intonation pattern.

A special use of intonation occurs for indicating sarcasm. The speaker uses a declarative statement, but with the intonation pattern of a question. For example:

That's a good idea.

The speaker's real meaning is: "You may think it's a good idea, but I don't," but in less confrontational wording.

RATE

We usually measure the **rate** at which speech is produced in the number of words or syllables per unit of time. The average duration of a syllable is 0.18 second. This corresponds to a rate of 5.0 to 5.5 syllables per second. In oral reading, most adults produce 150 to 180 words per minute. In actual conversational speech, you may produce 200 or more words per minute. Individuals vary, of course, in their speaking rate. The maximum rate of speech production appears to be influenced by articulatory control. We can improve our articulatory control (as evidenced by skillful speakers and debaters), but there is a limit to how much. For simple, repetitive articulatory movements, speakers reach a maximum rate of about 8 syllables per second. Even though the actual duration of different phonemes varies, you average a rate of 10 sounds per second in conversation. At 15 words per second, however, errors are frequent, and speech is distorted. On the other hand, speech understanding can occur at a much faster rate. So do silent reading and thinking. In fact, we can understand up to 30 sounds per second when paying careful attention.

Your speaking rate is influenced by a number of factors. The length and number of pauses, as well as the increased duration for stress and emphasis, all affect rate. Because stressed syllables have greater duration than unstressed, either habitual heavy stressing of syllables or great reduction on unstressed syllables will definitely influence overall speech rate. In normal conversation, the number of syllables in a phrase influences the rate. Thus, a speaker will take about the same amount of time to say "My name is Mary" and "My name is Mary Rich." The extra syllables get crammed in. This means that they must be spoken more rapidly. In difficult listening situations, you are more likely to reduce your speaking rate, using more and longer pauses. Understandability is also enhanced if you articulate more accurately, which also slows down the speaking rate. Additionally, emotion or mood can affect the rate. A tired, depressed person will probably speak at a slower rate, whereas an excited person will use a rapid rate, with syllables crammed together in short phrases.

There is no conventional way to mark rate visually. With IPA symbols, the curved underlined ligature can be used to show unusually rapid production. However, combining broad and narrow transcription together with markings for accent, emphasis, stressing, intonation, and rate requires highly skilled listening and transcription. Most likely, you would need to listen to a sample repeatedly to become accurate in the use of all these markings. Not surprisingly, most people use far fewer symbols in phonetic transcription. Often transcribing the phonemes and using narrow transcription symbols (see the first half of this chapter) will be sufficient for most purposes. Both narrow transcription symbols and markings for suprasegmental features can be very valuable in describing dialectic variations and speech disorders, the subjects covered in Chapters 8 and 9, respectively.

REVIEW VOCABULARY

accent   stress applied to a syllable in a word.

assimilation   conforming of one sound to the manner or place of articulation of a neighboring sound.

closed syllable   syllable ending in a consonant (e.g., CVC, VC).

coarticulation   influence of one speech sound upon a neighboring speech sound.

contiguous   referring to assimilation between phonemes directly adjacent to each other.

dentalization   shift in place of consonant articulation from alveolar to dental, due to presence of adjacent dental phonme (/θ/ or /ð/).

devoiced   loss of voicing for normally voiced phoneme due to assimilation.

diacritic markings   special transcription modification markers, used to indicate allophonic variations.

elision   one or a few consonants are omitted as a result of coarticulation.

emphasis   stress applied to a word in a phrase.

glottal stop   abrupt release of air at the glottis in connected speech.

haplology   omission of a whole syllable, typically occurring when two very similar syllables follow in close succession.

homorganic   made in the same place or with the same articulator position.

intervocalic voicing   voiceless singleton consonant becomes voiced between two vowels.

intonation   pitch variations within a phrase.

intonation contours   the pattern of pitch variations of intonation, including the degree, direction, and rate of pitch change.

juncture   transition point between words and phrases.

ligature   curved underlining to indicate phrasings.

nasal assimilation   nasal resonance of vowel resulting from proximity to a nasal consonant.

noncontiguous   referring to assimilation between phonemes separated by one or more other phonemes.

open syllable   syllable ending in a vowel (e.g., CV, CCV).

pause   silent intervals between phrases.

phonemic   having the characteristic of a phoneme by virtue of influencing the meaning of speech.

phrasing   organizing flowing speech into phrases.

progressive assimilation   change in phoneme characteristic(s) due to influence of a sound occurring earlier in the word.

rate   the number of syllables or words per unit of time.

regressive assimilation   change in phoneme characteristic(s) due to influence of a sound occurring later in the word.

segmental   referring to phoneme level of speech.

sonorant peak   speech segment of maximum energy in a syllable, typically a vowel.

sonority   refers to the relative loudness of speech sounds.

speech phrase   consists of a continuous utterance, bounded by silent intervals.

speech rhythm   general term referring to the combined aspects of accent, emphasis, phrasing, intonation, and rate.

stress   pointing up or drawing special attention to a speech unit.

suprasegmental aspects   speech features over and above phoneme segments, especially aspects of speech rhythm.

syllabic consonant   consonant that serves the function of a vowel as the nucleus of an unaccented syllable.

syllable   a cluster of coarticulated sounds with a single vowel or diphthong nucleus, with or without surrounding consonants.

trough   the portion of the syllable containing less energy than the sonorant peak (i.e., consonant(s)).

EXERCISES

CONNECTED SPEECH   Using the narrow transcription symbols you have learned, transcribe the following as you would say them in connected speech.

1. Voicing: [ˌ] [ˌ]

three	crew	behind	prey
sitting	little	slim	thrill
please	fry	ahead	butter

2. Lengthening: [:]

soon know	about time	bad days
some men	big glass	rib bones
full load	black car	ripe pears
spare ribs	top pots	this service

3. Syllabic consonants: []

little	ridden	bread 'n butter
kitten	bottle	riddle
cattle	Eden	cuddle
digging	meet 'em	driven

4. Intrusion: [t] [p] [k] [w] [j]

chance	something	go out	we each
no older	the east	strength	two hours
panther	comfort	to eat	no ID

5. Transcribe each of the following phrases in connected IPA transcription as you would say them in conversational speech. Each is a single phrase.

a. the easy way out
b. This seems OK.
c. better safe than sorry

SPEECH RHYTHM AND SUPRASEGMENTAL ASPECTS

6. Transcribe the following words in IPA symbols as you would say them, and mark the primary accent in each word.

natural   suspect (verb)   digital
inflation   suspect (noun)   reward
cobra   insult (verb)   tedious
video   insult (noun)   consenting

7. For the stressed word in the following repeated sentences, find the question/intent it signals to the listener.

Statement	Question/Intent
a. I'm too busy to handle that now.	I'm even busier than usual.
b. I'm too busy to handle that now.	I might have time later.
c. I'm too busy to handle that now.	All I could do is look at it, not deal with it.
d. I'm too busy to handle that now.	I could handle a smaller, different task.
e. I'm too busy to handle that now.	Someone else might be able to do it.

8. Transcribe the following speech units in connected IPA symbols as you (or another speaker) would say them, observing coarticulation effects, and marking phrasing and pause duration using /, //, and /// symbols.

a. I don't believe it. I got an A.
b. Oh, my. It's time to go.
c. Did you hear about that? I didn't.
d. They came in first and second, respectively.
e. Please bring me a pen, some paper, and a dictionary.

9. Indicate whether the following sentences would be characterized by rising, falling, or level intonation.

a. Are you coming?
b. I'm sorry.
c. I'm in here.
d. Who wants to know?
e. What's the difference?

CHAPTER 7

ACOUSTIC PHONETICS

BASIC CONCEPTS IN ACOUSTICS
GRAPHICAL REPRESENTATION OF ACOUSTIC SIGNALS
SPECTROGRAPHIC REPRESENTATION
THE NATURE OF SPEECH SOUNDS
VOWEL ACOUSTICS
ACOUSTIC NATURE OF SELECTED CONSONANTS
REVIEW VOCABULARY
EXERCISES

So far we have considered speech sounds mainly in terms of how we use our vocal mechanisms to produce them. Your study of phonetics would not be complete without an introduction to the acoustic nature of speech sounds. Our discussion in this text will be only an introduction. It is important for you to study the acoustic nature of speech sounds for several reasons. Acoustic analysis of speech sounds is rarely included in clinical processes or procedures. However, an understanding of speech acoustics will be very important for your understanding of the nature of communication disorders that are caused by hearing loss. Other applications of speech acoustics that have found use in clinical processes are machine synthesis of speech signals and automatic machine recognition of speech. Computers and computer-like devices can be programmed to produce synthetic speech signals and have found wide application in augmentative communication. In addition, speech recognition devices are finding applications in the speech-language clinic and other aspects of daily living. Both machine recognition of speech and machine synthesis of speech depend heavily on our understanding of the acoustic nature of speech signals.

In the following sections, we will consider basic acoustic parameters of speech sounds. We will consider first the basic fundamental principles of acoustic signals. It is customary for persons in communication sciences and disorders to represent acoustic signals graphically, rather than in mathematical equation form, so our discussion of basic principles will rely heavily on commonly used graphical formats. Discussion of graphical formats will culminate with the spectrogram, a graphical representation that allows us to represent the dynamic (time-varying) aspects of speech signals. Finally, we will use spectrographic analysis to illustrate the acoustic natures of various kinds of speech sounds.

BASIC CONCEPTS IN ACOUSTICS

Acoustic signals, commonly known as sound waves, are composed of more or less complicated vibrations of air particles, set into vibratory motion by some sort of acoustic source (a musical instrument or the human speech mechanism, for example). It is convenient to categorize acoustic signals into three broad categories, based on their patterns of vibration.

1. **Simple harmonic motion** (SHM; also called pure tones or sine waves) is the most basic form of acoustic energy. SHM rarely is heard by the human ear outside the laboratory because it is not commonly produced by anything in nature. However, it is an important building block of more complicated signals such as speech sounds.

2. **Complex harmonic motion** (CHM) is, as its name implies, a more complicated form of acoustic energy. As we will describe later in this chapter, complex harmonic motion signals are composed of two or more simple harmonic motion signals.

3. **Noise** is the third category of acoustic signal. Sounds categorized as noise are distinctly different from the harmonic signals in the first two categories in ways described below.

SIMPLE HARMONIC MOTION

Simple harmonic motion (SHM) is the simplest form of vibratory energy. It can be described as repetitive motion back and forth between two end points, with each back-and-forth cycle taking a specified amount of time. The **frequency** of a simple harmonic motion is the number of back-and-forth cycles per unit of time. The frequency of an SHM used to be measured in cycles per second. However, the modern term for cycles per second is **hertz,** abbreviated Hz. The normal adult human auditory system can hear SHM signals with frequency as low as about 20 Hz and as high as about 20,000 Hz. A signal with frequency of 20 Hz goes though 20 back-and-forth cycles each second. Similarly, a signal with frequency of 20,000 Hz completes 20,000 cycles each second. Generally, SHM signals with lower frequency are heard as lower in pitch, and higher frequency signals are perceived as higher in pitch. (Musically, low-frequency and high-frequency sounds are heard as base and treble, respectively.)

One way to visualize a simple harmonic motion is to imagine a Slinky suspended from one end, with the other end hanging free. Imagine hanging a small weight on the free end of the Slinky. Now imagine that the weight is pulled downward momentarily, then released. It will immediately travel upward toward and past its original position. It will then continue in a regular pattern of up-and-down movement between two end points that are equidistant from the original resting position. The motion of the weight on the Slinky will be very close to SHM, except much slower than that of acoustic signals. You could count the number of up-and-down excursions of the weight in each second. The number of cycles per second would be the frequency of the SHM. Another important characteristic of SHM is its **amplitude,** or the distance between the end points of its vibratory pattern. Magnitude (of motion) might be another way to think of amplitude. In acoustic signals, the human ear perceives amplitude primarily as loudness; that is, acoustic signals with smaller amplitude generally are perceived as softer sounds. Conversely, acoustic signals with higher amplitude are perceived as louder.

The term *simple harmonic motion,* then, can be broken down in this way:

- *Simple* refers to the simple back-and-forth pattern of vibration between two end points, which are equidistant from the resting position of the vibratory object.
- *Harmonic* refers to the pattern of vibration that repeats at regular intervals in time.
- *Motion* refers to some physical object that is in motion.

Thus, vibration characterized by a vibratory object moving back-and-forth between two end points in a pattern that repeats itself in regular time intervals is called simple harmonic motion.

COMPLEX HARMONIC MOTION

Complex harmonic motion (CHM) is a very large family of vibratory patterns. Similar to SHM, CHM signals have regular vibratory patterns that are repeated at regular, or **harmonic,** intervals in time. However, their vibratory patterns are more involved. All CHM signals are composed of two or more simple harmonic motion components. Indeed, the vowel sounds of speech are CHM signals, and they are composed of a large number of SHM components. With the exception of much of the percussion family, musical instruments produce complex harmonic motion. When you set a guitar string in motion by plucking, the string vibrates in a complex harmonic motion pattern and produces a sound wave identical to the pattern of vibration of the string. Likewise, the brass and woodwind instruments produce complex harmonic motion sounds. Because they are CHM sounds, they are composed of many simple harmonic motion components, all added together.

The SHM components in a complex harmonic motion are called **harmonics.** Harmonics of a CHM are related to each other by constant frequency intervals. The interval between harmonics in a CHM is called its **fundamental frequency.** An average adult male, sustaining any vowel sound, produces a complex harmonic motion sound that has a fundamental frequency of approximately 100 Hz and would have SHM components (harmonics) at intervals of 100 Hz. That is, it would have harmonics at frequencies of 100, 200, 300, 400, 500 Hz, and so on, through at least 6000 Hz. An average adult female who vocalizes the same vowel typically would have a fundamental frequency of about 200 Hz. Therefore, the SHM components (harmonics) that comprise this sound would be at intervals of 200 Hz (200, 400, 600, 800 Hz, and so, on through at least 6000 Hz).

NOISE

Noise is the third classification of acoustic signals. Sounds are classified as noise if they are not harmonic.[1] Therefore, sounds classified as noise are not characterized

---

[1]The word *noise* has several meanings in English usage. Here, we use it to refer to acoustic signals that are not harmonic; that is, sounds that do not have vibratory patterns characterized by repetition at regular intervals in time. We often use the word *noise* as a synonym for the word *sound.* This is perfectly acceptable in everyday use. However, in our study of speech acoustics, the two words, *sound* and *noise,* have two very different meanings. The word *sound* refers to any acoustic signal, SHM, CHM, or noise, whereas the word *noise* refers specifically to sounds that are not harmonic.

by patterns that are repeated in regular time intervals. Noise signals are characterized by random, or quasi-random, changes in displacement as a function of time. Signals characterized as noise do not have harmonics at regular frequency intervals. Noise signals that can be sustained for long periods of time are called continuous noises. In speech, fricative sounds such as [s] and [ʃ] are continuous noises. Noises that cannot be sustained for a long duration (very brief noises) are called transient noises. A single firecracker will generate a transient noise. A single hand clap is another example of a transient noise. Transient noises are also found in speech. For example, the very brief burst of energy associated with the release of a voiceless stop consonant is a transient noise.

GRAPHICAL REPRESENTATION OF ACOUSTIC SIGNALS

We use three different types of graphics to represent acoustic signals: (1) waveform; (2) spectrum, which can be either line spectrum or spectrum envelope; and (3) spectrogram. These will be illustrated in the next several sections.

Figure 7–1 illustrates an example of the **waveform** (form of the wave) of an SHM. Amplitude is shown on the vertical axis, as a function of time, which is represented on the horizontal axis. This illustration shows 10 complete cycles of a simple harmonic motion. The physical motion represented in this figure is simply back and forth between two end points, +A and −A on the vertical axis. The horizontal axis represents time, from earlier to later. Panels A and B in Figure 7–2 represent SHM waveforms that differ from each other only with respect to frequency. The SHM in the top panel has a frequency of 1000 Hz. Notice that there are 10 complete cycles in a time interval of 0.01 second. Because each individual cycle requires 0.001 second, the signal frequency must be 1000 Hz. Panel B represents an SHM frequency of 500 Hz. Note that there are only five complete cycles of the waveform in the same 0.01 second time interval, so each individual cycle requires 0.002 second to complete.

If two or more SHM signals are added together under the proper conditions, the result will be a complex harmonic signal. Panel C in Figure 7–2 represents a complex harmonic signal comprising the two signals in Panels A and B of Figure 7–2. That is, when we add a 500 Hz SHM to a 1000 Hz SHM of equal amplitude, we get the CHM signal shown in Panel C. It is important for you to notice that this motion is not simply back and forth between two end points. Rather, the pattern of vibration is such that it has minor negative and positive peaks (indicated by the arrows in Figure 7–2) between the positive end point and the negative end point. Also, please notice that the period of this CHM is the same as the period of the interval between the SHM components, 500 Hz.

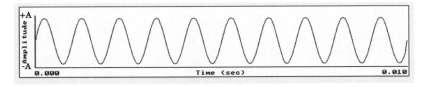

Figure 7–1 *Waveform representation of 10 cycles of a 1000 Hz simple harmonic motion (SHM) signal. The waveform represents displacement of a vibratory object (on the vertical axis) as a function of time (on the horizontal axis). In this example, the SHM is back and forth between points +A and −A on the vertical axis.*

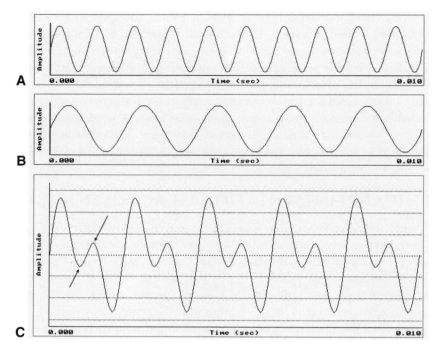

Figure 7–2 *The top two panels contain waveform representations of SHM signals with frequencies of 1000 Hz (Panel A) and 500 Hz (Panel B). Panel C contains a waveform representation of a complex harmonic motion (CHM) signal, the additive combination of the SHM signals in Panels A and B. The arrows point to minor positive and negative peaks between the positive and negative major peaks.*

The CHM in Figure 7–2 is composed of only two SHM components. Most natural examples of CHM are composed of many more than two components. A vowel sound, for example, is composed of dozens of simple harmonic motion components, all added together to produce a very intricate form of complex harmonic motion. Examples can be seen in Figures 7–7 and 7–8.

Finally, Figure 7–3 represents the waveform of a 0.01 second sample of a continuous noise. The distinguishing characteristic of this kind of signal is that it is not **periodic.** That is, the vibratory motion is not characterized by a pattern that is repeated at regular intervals in time. Rather, the motion can be described as random direction and speed. Therefore, continuous noise of this sort can also be called **random noise.**

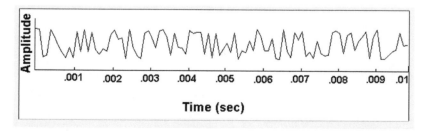

Figure 7–3 *Waveform representation of a 0.01 second sample of a noise signal. Note that this signal is not harmonic; it is not characterized by a vibratory pattern that is repeated at regular intervals in time.*

Another graphic that is often used to represent acoustic signals is the spectrum, which can take the form of either a line spectrum or a spectrum envelope. **Spectrum** representation of acoustic signals is also a two-dimensional graphic, this time with frequency on the horizontal axis and amplitude on the vertical axis. Lower frequency signals are represented toward the left, and higher frequency signals are represented toward the right. Smaller amplitude signals are represented by short lines; conversely, larger amplitude signals are represented by longer lines. (Note that time is not represented on a spectrum.) Figure 7–4 contains line spectra for the signals used in previous examples (500 Hz and 1000 Hz SHM, the CHM from Figure 7–2, and a noise). The 500 Hz (Panel A) and 1000 Hz (Panel B) SHM examples are represented by a vertical line drawn to the horizontal axis from the point of intersect of frequency and amplitude. Each of the two examples of SHM is represented by a single line. Panel A represents a 500 Hz SHM so it is located at the 500 Hz point on the horizontal axis. Similarly, the 1000 Hz SHM in Panel B is located at the 1000 Hz point on the horizontal axis. Notice in Panel C we must use two lines to represent the two SHM components of the CHM produced by adding the 500 Hz and 1000 Hz signals together. Finally, the noise represented by

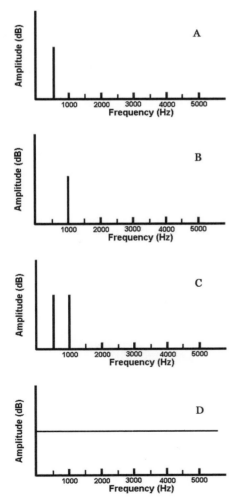

Figure 7–4 Spectrum representations of a 500 Hz SHM (Panel A), 1000 Hz SHM (Panel B), CHM consisting of two SHM components (Panel C), and a continuous noise (Panel D).

the spectrum in Figure 7–4 (Panel D) looks as if it does not have any lines. Actually, the lines are so close together that there are no spaces between them. That is, the noise has components at each and every frequency in the spectrum. Because it is not composed of harmonics at discrete frequency intervals, it is not harmonic and has no fundamental frequency.

SPECTROGRAPHIC REPRESENTATION

So far we have described two kinds of graphic representation of acoustic signals: (1) the waveform, with amplitude on the vertical axis plotted against time on the horizontal axis, and (2) spectrum, with amplitude on the vertical axis plotted against frequency on the horizontal axis. Of these two, we are able to represent more information about complex harmonic motion with the spectrum. With the spectrum, however, we are not able to represent changes in an acoustic signal that take place over time. Because the acoustic signals in speech change rapidly over time, we need a spectrum-like representation that will enable us to represent the acoustic signal at various points in time. We can achieve this with a graphic representation called the **spectrogram.** Spectrogram representations plot frequency along the vertical axis, with time represented along the horizontal axis. Amplitude is represented by the darkness of the mark, with higher amplitude signals represented by darker lines and lower amplitude signals represented by lines that are less dark. Figure 7–5 depicts the spectrographic representation of a sine wave that is changing in frequency. Time is on the horizontal axis, progressing from earlier (toward the left) to later in time (toward the right). The vertical axis represents frequency in 500 Hz increments, from 0 to 4000 Hz. Look at Figure 7–5 and verify that the acoustic signal represented here begins (toward the left) as a 500 Hz sine wave, and that the frequency of this signal changes over time until it ends as a 3000 Hz signal. (Starting and ending frequencies are identified for you.) The amplitude of this signal remains constant, as indicated by the constant darkness. A smaller amplitude (softer) signal would be lighter, and a higher amplitude (louder) signal would be darker.

Spectrographic representation is a very important tool for learning about and understanding the acoustic nature of speech sounds. Most of the illustrations in the remainder of this chapter will rely on spectrographic representation.

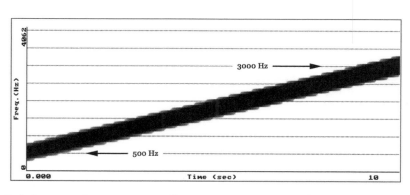

Figure 7–5 *Spectrographic representation of an SHM signal that changes frequency, beginning at 500 Hz and ending at 3000 Hz. The beginning and ending frequencies are marked with arrows.*

THE NATURE OF SPEECH SOUNDS

The speech production apparatus can be considered as two separate (but certainly connected) mechanisms, the voice production apparatus (lungs and larynx) and the vocal tract (pharynx, oral cavity, and nasal cavity). During speech production, the vocal tract acts as a **resonator** to modify the sound source produced at the larynx.

THE LARYNGEAL SOURCE

During phonation, the larynx opens and closes very rapidly, producing a buzzlike sound. For an average-size adult male, the rate of opening and closing of the vocal folds is approximately 100 Hz; that is, the vocal folds open and close about 100 times each second. This would be a fundamental frequency of 100 Hz. For an adult female, the rate is about twice as fast, about 200 times each second, which would be a complex harmonic motion with fundamental frequency of 200 Hz. We can never hear the buzzlike sound that comes directly from the larynx because it is always modified by the resonances of the vocal tract. However, we know the acoustic signal produced by the larynx is a complex harmonic motion with fundamental frequency equal to the rate of opening and closing of the vocal folds. The acoustic spectrum of the laryngeal source is represented in Figure 7–6. Notice that the fundamental frequency represented in Figure 7–6 is 100 Hz because the harmonics are spaced at 100 Hz intervals, from 100 Hz to 3000 Hz. A laryngeal source produced by a typical adult female would have harmonics spaced at intervals of about 200 Hz, beginning with 200 Hz.

We can change the nature of the laryngeal source in only two ways: fundamental frequency and amplitude. We can change fundamental frequency by making the vocal folds more or less rigid. More rigid vocal folds will vibrate faster and therefore produce a higher fundamental frequency. Conversely, less rigid vocal folds will vibrate more slowly and produce a lower fundamental frequency. Perceptually,

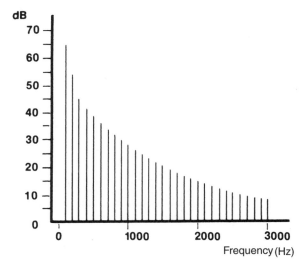

Figure 7–6 Line spectrum of an idealized glottal sound with fundamental frequency of 100 Hz. This is the spectrum of the sound produced by the larynx, before it goes through the vocal tract. This would sound like a buzz, if we could hear it.

changes in fundamental frequency are heard as changes in intonation. Therefore, intonation is a vocal characteristic that we control with the larynx. We can also change the amplitude of the laryngeal source by altering the air pressure from the lungs. More air pressure produces higher signal amplitude, and less air pressure produces lower amplitudes. We hear changes in amplitude as changes in stress. Therefore, we can surmise that both stress and intonation are produced by changes we make at the level of the larynx.

VOCAL TRACT RESONANCES

The buzzlike signal produced by the larynx must pass though the vocal tract before it exits the speech production apparatus. The vocal tract is a complicated system of resonances that can be varied by changing the shape of the vocal tract. The spectral shape of the laryngeal signal is modified as it travels through the vocal tract resonances. That is, the spectrum of the laryngeal source is shaped by the resonances of the vocal tract. If the vocal tract of an average adult male is held in a posture that most closely resembles a straight tube, it would have resonances at frequencies of 500, 1500, 2500, and 3500 Hz. In passing through the vocal tract, harmonics in the laryngeal source that are close to the resonant frequencies would be enhanced, and harmonics at frequencies between the resonances would be reduced in amplitude. The result would be the spectrum shown in Figure 7–7. Comparing Figures 7–6 and 7–7 will confirm that harmonics close to the resonant frequencies of the vocal tract (500, 1500, and 2500 Hz) have been enhanced and that the spectrum of the laryngeal source has been shaped by the resonances of the vocal tract. Figure 7–8 provides another example; this one represents the acoustic spectrum that would result if a typical adult male sustained the vowel /i/. Notice that the lowest frequency resonance is near the third harmonic, about 300 Hz in this example. The next resonances are between 2000 and 3000 Hz.

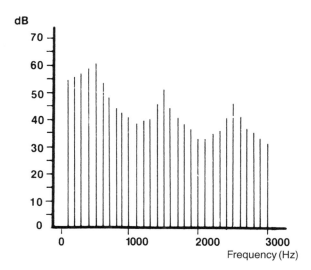

Figure 7–7 Line spectrum that would result if the laryngeal source went through and was shaped by an idealized vocal tract. An idealized vocal tract would have the shape of a straight cylindrical tube. If the tube is 17 cm long (the length of an average adult male vocal tract), it would have resonant frequencies of 500, 1500, and 2500 Hz.

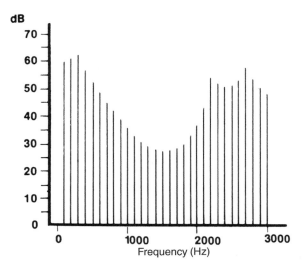

Figure 7–8 *Line spectrum that would result if the laryngeal source went through and was shaped by an average adult male vocal tract held in a posture that would produce the high-front vowel /i/.*

Resonances in the vocal tract shape the laryngeal source, augmenting the amplitudes of harmonics that are near the resonances. In the resulting acoustic signal, spectral areas that have been augmented by the resonances are called formants. **Formants** are numbered from low to high so that the first formant is the one that occurs at the lowest frequency. Thus, in Figure 7–8, the first formant is at 300 Hz, the second is at 2200 Hz, and the third is at 2700 Hz. (When you try to verify the first three formant frequencies of Figure 7–8, remember that the fundamental frequency is 100 Hz, so that harmonics are spaced evenly at intervals of 100 Hz. Because harmonics are evenly spaced at 100 Hz intervals, you can determine the frequency of any particular harmonic by counting by 100s from the first harmonic.)

VOWEL ACOUSTICS

As you have already learned, vowels are differentiated from each other on the physical bases of at least (1) **tongue height,** (2) **tongue advancement,** and (3) lip rounding. Here, the term *tongue advancement* refers to the location in the vocal tract (front to back) of the constriction formed by the tongue and the hard palate. Recall from Chapters 3 and 4 that /i/, /ɪ/, /e/, /ɛ/, and /æ/ are front vowels because the tongue is relatively forward during their production. Similarly, /ɑ/, /ɔ/, /o/, /ʊ/, and /u/ are back vowels because the tongue is relatively far back in the vocal tract during their production. The term *tongue height* refers to the degree of constriction formed by the tongue and the hard palate. Higher tongue postures create narrower construction, as required for the high vowels /i/, /ɪ/, /ʊ/, and /u/. Conversely, lower tongue postures create less vocal tract constriction, as required for the low vowels /ɛ/, /æ/, /ɑ/, and /ɔ/. Finally, lip rounding is required for most of the back vowels. Recall from Chapters 3 and 4 that /ɑ/ is the only back vowel that does not require lip rounding.

We know that each of these physical dimensions has an influence on the acoustic nature of the vowels. That is, vowels produced with different tongue height differ from each other acoustically, as do vowels that differ from each other in tongue advancement. Lip rounding also has a distinct influence on the acoustic signal that is produced. Different tongue heights are illustrated in Figure 4–1 (front vowels) and Figure 4–2 (back vowels). High vowels are produced with a high tongue posture, resulting in relatively narrow constriction. On the other hand, low vowels are produced with a low tongue posture, resulting in less constriction of the vocal tract. The acoustical properties associated with the various vowel postures are described in the next sections.

TONGUE ADVANCEMENT

First, second, and third formant frequencies of selected vowels are represented in Figure 7–9. Refer to this figure often as you read the following text. Tongue height, the degree of constriction formed by the tongue as it approximates the hard palate, is most closely related to the frequency of the first format. When we produce a vowel with narrow construction (tongue held high in the vocal tract), the first formant of the vowel is a relatively low frequency. When we produce vowels with wider constrictions (the tongue held low in the vocal tract), we produce vowels with higher first formant frequency. Now, go to Figure 7–9 and verify that the two vowels with the lowest first formant frequency are /i/ and /u/, the two highest vowels. Both /i/ and /u/ have a first formant frequency of about 250 Hz (about halfway between 0 and 500 Hz on the vertical axis). Notice also that the two lowest vowels, /æ/ and /ɑ/, have the highest first formant frequencies. First formant of /æ/ is about 600 Hz, and first formant for /ɑ/ is closer to 750 Hz (halfway between 500 and 1000 Hz on the vertical axis).

TONGUE HEIGHT

Just as the first formant is most closely related to tongue height, the second formant is most closely related to tongue advancement, particularly for the front vowels. Notice in Figure 7–9 that the second formant is always a higher frequency for the front vowels and a lower frequency for the back vowels. In fact, there is a very orderly progression of second formant frequency from /i/ through /æ/, with progressively lower second formant frequency for lower vowels. For the back vowels, lip rounding tends to reduce the frequencies of both first and second formants.

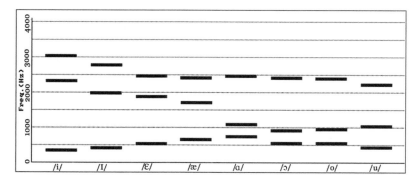

Figure 7–9 *Approximate average formant frequencies (for the first three formants) for the average adult male vocal tract.*

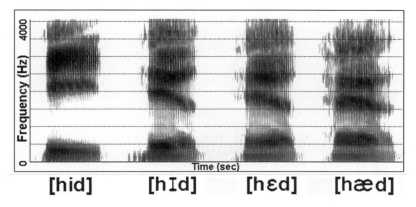

Figure 7–10 *Spectrographic representation of four syllables containing four front vowels.*

Figure 7–10 shows the spectrographic analysis of four front vowels. Spectrograms of four back vowels are shown in Figure 7–11. Take the time to identify the first and second formant frequencies for each of the eight vowels in these figures, and compare them with the formant frequencies given in Figure 7–9.

ACOUSTIC NATURE OF SELECTED CONSONANTS

Certain acoustic features that differentiate the various categories of consonants can best be illustrated by spectrographic representation. In the illustrations that follow, we will use only prevocalic consonants. In the first sections, we will consider the more obvious acoustic nature of selected consonants. Then, in later sections, we will focus on the acoustic distinctions among selected articulatory features of consonants.

STOP CONSONANTS

Recall that stop consonants are produced by complete closure of the vocal tract, which, at least for prevocalic stops, is followed by an abrupt release. In many prevocalic stops, release of the stop closure usually is associated with a brief explosion of air, or plosive. The plosive portion of a stop consonant can be seen clearly in Figure

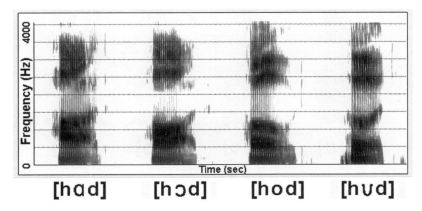

Figure 7–11 *Spectrographic representation of four syllables containing four back vowels.*

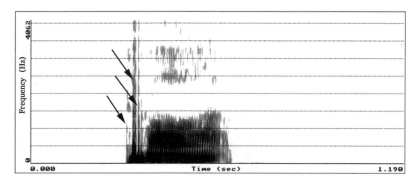

Figure 7–12 *Spectrographic representation of the syllable /tɔt/ (taught). The arrows point to the impulse noise associated with the plosive portion of the initial consonant /t/. Note that the final /t/ is not released.*

7–12, which is a spectrographic analysis of the syllable, /tɔt/ (*taught*). The arrows point to the impulse noise associated with the plosive portion of this consonant. Stop consonants are not always released in postvocalic contexts. That is, when a stop consonant is produced at the end of a phrase, it is not released, so there is no noise burst. Rather, final stop consonants in postvocalic, syllable-final, contexts are cued only by the rate and direction of the formant transitions (as will be described later in the chapter). You can see in Figure 7–12 that there is no noise burst associated with the final /t/ as there is with the initial /t/.

FRICATIVE CONSONANTS

Fricative consonants are produced by forcing a stream of air through a very narrow opening in the vocal tract, which produces a turbulent flow of air. Air turbulence is simply noise as we defined it earlier in this chapter. Figure 7–13 shows four consonant-vowel syllables with each of four voiceless fricative initial consonants. The noise associated with each of the consonants is indicated by the arrows. Notice that the noise portion is of very short duration and somewhat difficult to identify

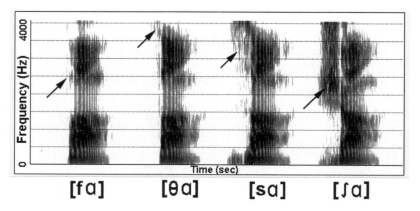

Figure 7–13 *Spectrographic representation of four syllables containing four different syllable-initial fricative consonants. The arrows point to the fricative noise positions of each consonant. Note that the noises associated with /s/ and /ʃ/ are more prominent than the noises associated with /f/ and /θ/.*

for /f/ and /θ/. In contrast, the consonants /s/ and /ʃ/ have longer duration and higher amplitude, making them easier to identify. Indeed, studies of consonant intelligibility indicate that the latter two consonants are easier for people to identify than are the former two. The distinctions have led some linguists to differentiate between the sibilant (/s/-colored) fricatives and the nonsibilant fricatives. The higher amplitude of the noise associated with sibilant fricatives is related to the airstream crossing the cutting edge of the upper front teeth, an action that creates additional turbulence.

LIQUIDS AND GLIDES

Liquids and glides are characterized acoustically by their striking similarities to vowels and vowel-like sounds. Their similarity to vowels and vowel-like sounds is attributed to the fact that liquids and glides are produced with relatively little vocal tract constriction. Figure 7–14 shows two consonant-vowel syllables, /jɑ/ and /wɑ/. The consonantal portion of each syllable is indicated with the arrows and brackets at the top of the spectrogram. Notice that the rapid changes in first and second formant frequency are the result of the gliding gestures of vocal tract posture. (Second formant starting and ending frequencies are indicated by the horizontal arrows.) That is, in order to produce a glide, we move our vocal tract from the initial posture to the posture associated with the vowel nucleus in a smooth gliding pattern. Formant frequencies change as the vocal tract posture changes during the production of these consonants.

VOICING

The acoustic distinction between voiced and voiceless consonants depends on consonant classification and is different for fricatives than for stop consonants. The voicing distinction for fricative consonants depends only on whether voice is produced during the frication portion of the syllable. For example, voicing is not used during the production of the voiceless /f/; however, voicing is used for production of the voiced cognate, /v/. The contrast can be seen in Figure 7–15, which shows the acoustic distinction between /fɑ/ and /vɑ/. The voicing distinction between

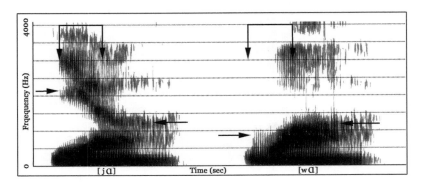

Figure 7–14 *Spectrographic representation of two syllables with syllable-initial glide consonants /j/ and /w/. The consonant-to-vowel formant transitions are marked with vertical arrows and brackets. Right-pointing arrows indicate approximate starting frequency for second formant transitions, and left-pointing arrows indicate the midsyllable frequencies for first and second formants.*

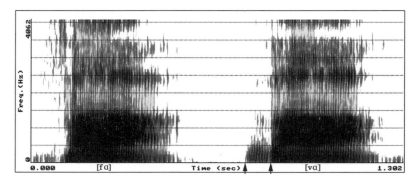

Figure 7–15 Spectrographic representation of two syllables, /fɑ/ and /vɑ/. The voicing bar, indicative of a voiced fricative, is indicated by the arrows at the bottom of the spectrogram.

these two syllable-initial consonants can be seen best at the bottom of the spectrograms. Notice that for the voiced /v/, we see a dark, low-frequency bar preceding the syllable nucleus. This "voicing bar" indicates the presence of low-frequency energy associated with voicing during the frication portion of the syllable. Contrast this with the lack of a "voicing bar" during the frication portion of the syllable /fɑ/. You will notice vertical striations in the voicing bar associated with the voiced fricative. This regular vertical striation pattern is associated with individual cycles of the laryngeal source and serves as a positive indicator of voicing.

The voicing distinction for stop consonants is just a little more complicated. We will consider it in relation to prevocalic stop consonants; these observations can easily be extrapolated for postvocalic and intervocalic stop consonants. Recall that the production of stop consonants requires the vocal tract to be completely closed for a brief period (the stop closure). The voicing feature of stop consonants is determined by the relative timing of the onset of voicing in relation to the point in time when the stop closure is released. The distinction can be illustrated by the contrast in Figure 7–16 which shows spectrograms of /tɑ/ on the left and /dɑ/ on

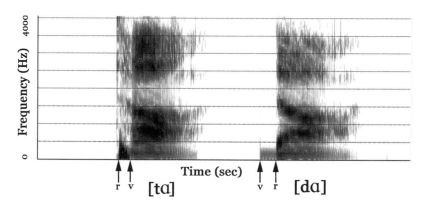

Figure 7–16 Spectographic representation of two syllables, /tɑ/ and /dɑ/. The onset of voicing is indicated by "v" and the release of the stop is indicated by "r" along the horizontal axis. Notice in the syllable, /tɑ/, the stop is released before the onset of voicing. However, in the syllable, /dɑ/, the onset of voicing occurs before the stop is released.

the right. The moment of voicing onset is indicated by *v* on the horizontal axis. Similarly, the moment when the stop closure is released is shown by *r* on the horizontal axis. In the spectrogram of /tɑ/, notice that the stop release and its associated brief noise burst precede the onset of voicing. However, in order to produce the syllable /dɑ/, voicing must be initiated before the stop closure is released. Be aware that one can barely sustain voicing with a completely closed vocal tract, so release of the stop closure for a voiced stop consonant must happen a very small fraction of a second after the onset of voicing. The phenomenon just illustrated is called voice onset time (VOT). Officially, VOT is the amount of time measured from stop release to voice onset. VOT is a positive value for voiceless stops and a negative value for voiced stops.

PLACE OF ARTICULATION

The place of articulation feature of most consonants is manifest acoustically by changes in formant frequencies that result from changes in vocal tract posture. The acoustic phenomenon of formant transitions can be seen most easily in voiced stop consonants. Figure 7–17 contains spectrographic representation of the syllables /bɑ/, /dɑ/, and /gɑ/. Formant transitions are indicated by the arrows and brackets at the top of the spectrogram. Formant transition starting frequencies are indicated by right-pointing arrows. First and second formant frequencies for the vowel nucleus are indicated by left-pointing arrows. In each syllable, the first vertical arrow marks the onset of the formant transition, and the second vertical arrow marks the end of the transition. Look at the second formant for the syllable /bɑ/. The second formant begins at approximately 1000 Hz and ends, midsyllable, at about 1200 Hz. At the moment the stop portion of the consonant is broken, the vocal tract is in a posture that produces a second resonance of about 1000 Hz. Then, immediately after the stop portion is broken, the vocal tract posture moves rapidly toward the posture appropriate for the vowel nucleus. Once the posture for the vowel nucleus is achieved, the second formant frequency is about 1200 Hz. So, for the consonant-vowel syllable /bɑ/, the bilabial place of articulation results in a

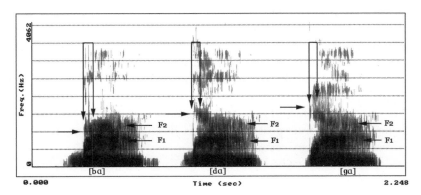

Figure 7–17 *Spectrographic representation of three syllables with syllable-initial stop consonants /b/, /d/, and /g/. The consonant-to-vowel formant transitions are marked with vertical arrows and brackets. Right-pointing arrows indicate approximate starting frequency for second formant transitions, and left-pointing arrows indicate the midsyllable frequencies for first and second formants.*

rapid second formant transition from 1000 to 1200 Hz (marked with horizontal arrows). Now look at the second formant transition associated with the syllable /dɑ/. The second formant in /bɑ/ begins at approximately 1500 Hz and ends with the vowel nucleus, again at approximately 1200 Hz. Finally, observe that the starting frequency for the second formant in the syllable /gɑ/ is about 1700 Hz. An important acoustic difference between these two syllables, therefore, is in the starting frequency of the second formant. This is a major acoustic cue that we use to identify the place of articulation in many consonants. Formant transitions for stop consonants take about 0.04 second to accomplish in natural fluent speech. As vocal tract posture moves from consonant to vowel nucleus posture, all formants change in frequency.

Another illustration of the importance of formant transitions in production and perception of place of articulation can be seen in the final /t/ shown in Figure 7–12. Recall, that syllable-final stop consonants often are produced without release of the stop. If you examine the second formant of the syllable, /tɔt, in Figure 7–12, from syllabic nucleus to the end of the syllable, you will see that the second formant increases in frequency toward the end of the syllable. This upward second formant transition is the only obvious cue for identification of place of articulation for this final /t/.

We have focused on the second formant in this illustration because the second formant is the single most important acoustic cue for perception of place of articulation, particularly for stop, nasal, and glide consonants.

MANNER OF ARTICULATION

The clearest distinction in manner of articulation is between stop and glide consonants. Compare the consonant-to-vowel transitions for the two bilabial consonants in Figures 7–14 (/wɑ/) and 7–17 (/bɑ/). Both of these consonants are considered as having a bilabial place of articulation. Therefore, they both are produced with vocal tract movements from bilabial posture to the posture appropriate for the vowel nucleus. Careful inspection of the two spectrograms will confirm that second formants for both /bɑ/ and /wɑ/ begin at 1000 Hz or less and end in the vowel nucleus at about 1200 Hz (as indicated by the horizontal arrows). The difference between them is related to the amount of time required to produce the consonant-to-vowel transition. As already indicated, the formant transitions for stop consonants take about 0.04 second to articulate because the vocal tract is moving very rapidly from one posture to another. On the other hand, the formant transitions for glide consonants require much more time, as long as 0.1 second, because articulators are moving more slowly. Stop consonants are produced with rapid and abrupt changes in vocal tract posture, whereas glide consonants are produced with slower "gliding" articulatory gestures.

Obviously, we have described the acoustic nature of only a few selected consonants and consonantal features because this was intended only as an introduction to acoustic phonetics. Equally important are the acoustic characteristics of other consonant classifications, such as affricates and nasals. The student of phonetics is encouraged to continue exploration of the acoustic nature of speech sounds as it relates to (1) the link between articulator posture and the acoustic nature of speech sounds and (2) the acoustic cues we use in speech perception to identify the various sounds of speech.

REVIEW VOCABULARY

amplitude   the magnitude of an acoustic signal; how far a vibratory object travels in its pattern of vibration.

complex harmonic motion   a vibratory pattern that is repeated at regular intervals in time; complex harmonic motion always is composed of two or more simple harmonic motion signals (called harmonics) added together.

formant   a resonance in the vocal tract that enhances harmonics (in the laryngeal source) that are near the resonant frequency.

frequency   the number of cycles of a vibratory pattern per unit of time; in acoustics, frequency is measured in cycles per second, also called hertz.

fundamental frequency   the interval, in hertz, between any two adjacent harmonics in a complex harmonic motion signal.

harmonic (periodic)   a sound that is harmonic has a systematic pattern of vibration that is repeated at regular time intervals.

harmonics   simple harmonic motion components that, when added together, join to make a complex harmonic motion; each simple harmonic motion component is called a harmonic.

hertz   frequency of vibratory motion is measured in hertz (Hz); the number of vibratory cycles per second.

noise   any acoustic signal that is not harmonic; an acoustic signal not characterized by a repetitive vibratory pattern.

periodic (harmonic)   a sound that is harmonic has a systematic pattern of vibration that is repeated at regular time intervals.

random noise   a nonharmonic signal with vibratory pattern characterized by random (or quasi-random) direction and speed.

resonator   an acoustic device that vibrates better at its natural frequency than other frequencies; a resonator augments signals that are close to its natural frequency and reduces the amplitude of signals that are not close to its natural frequency.

simple harmonic motion   vibratory motion characterized by a simple pattern, back and forth between two end points, and that repeats itself at regular intervals in time.

spectrogram   graphic representation of acoustic signals, with frequency on the vertical axis and time on the horizontal axis.

spectrum   graphic representation of acoustic signals, with amplitude on the vertical axis and frequency on the horizontal axis.

tongue advancement   in vowel articulation, the location (front-to-back) of the major constriction formed with the tongue.

tongue height   in vowel articulation, the height of the major constriction formed by the tongue.

waveform   graphic representation of acoustic signals, with amplitude on the vertical axis and time on the horizontal axis.

EXERCISES

1. Figure 7–9 provides a graphic representation of the formant frequencies for the first three formants (F1, F2, and F3) of eight vowels. In this exercise, you are to estimate the first three formant frequencies from Figure 7–9 and complete Table 7–1 below.

   To get you started, go to Figure 7–9 and look at the leftmost vowel, /i/. Notice that the first formant for this vowel is approximately 300 Hz, a little more than halfway between 0 and 500 Hz. You determine this by locating the black bar that represents the first formant (the lowest frequency formant) and reading the formant frequency on the vertical axis. The first formant frequency for /i/ (300 Hz) is already inserted in the table. Now, find the approximate second and third formant frequencies for /i/ from Figure 7–9. (They should be about 2400 Hz and 3100 Hz, respectively.) Write these in the appropriate spaces (in the column headed /i/) in Table 7–1. Now, complete the remainder of the table. Remember, you are finding only the approximate formant frequencies.

TABLE 7–1 APPROXIMATE FORMANT FREQUENCIES FOR THE FIRST THREE FORMANTS (F1, F2, F3) FOR EIGHT SELECTED VOWELS

	/i/	/ɪ/	/ɛ/	/æ/	/ɑ/	/ɔ/	/o/	/u/
F1	300 Hz							
F2								
F3								

CHAPTER 8

MULTICULTURAL VARIATIONS: DIALECTS

DEFINITIONS
DIFFERENT VIEWS OF DIALECT
SOURCES OF DIALECTIC VARIATION
REVIEW VOCABULARY
EXERCISES

DEFINITIONS

Throughout this book we have presented word pronunciations characteristic of what has been referred to in earlier texts as **standard American English (SAE)** or **general American English (GAE).** Another term sometimes used is **mainstream English (ME),** particularly by professionals who study and work with a variety of regional or cultural dialect speakers. In general, ME is supposed to be relatively free of any distinctively regional characteristics (Wolfram, 1991). How do we decide what is "mainstream"? Typically, the English pronunciation and grammar used in textbooks and school instruction has been the source for what is mainstream. National television broadcasters also usually provide an example of what would be called ME. In general, these pronunciations and grammar usage are understood by the widest possible number of Americans. Most often, this means that the English spoken in the Midwest and central regions of the United States tends to be the model for ME. Obviously, if you are from the South **(Southern English, or SE)** or **New England (NEE),** you know that your pronunciation varies in some ways from ME. For example, in both these regional dialects, speakers omit or neutralize postvocalic /ɹ/. Thus, *park the car* [p ɑ r k ð ə k ɑ r] in ME becomes [p ɑ ək ð ə k ɑ ə] or [p ɑ:k ð ə k ɑ:] in these dialects. This chapter will introduce you to dialects and their transcription.

We begin by discussing key terms for this chapter. There are two terms for you to understand: *dialect* and *accent*. Although the definitions can vary, we will follow the manner of several professional associations (Montgomery, 1999). **Dialect** refers to a set of differences that make the speech of one English speaker different from another's (Montgomery, 1999; Wolfram & Fasold, 1974). These differences can include phonological, morphological, and grammatical differences. Although American English dialects do differ, the vast majority of their characteristics are the same. (That is why you can usually understand someone who speaks a different dialect, although you may have to get used to the way they sound.) **Accent** most often refers to the phonetic and suprasegmental traits that characterize a person's speech. Thus, accent is concerned with fewer features of a person's speech than is dialect. Typically, what the ME speaker notices in NEE is related to accent or pronunciation changes. As we noted earlier, ME uses full pronunciation of /ɹ/ in all word positions; NEE does not. In addition, NEE speakers use what is referred to as a broad *a* or /a/. This pronunciation occurs in words like *half* and *calf*, in which ME speakers would use /æ/.

Dialect variations affecting vocabulary can be found in a number of words. Depending on your dialect, you will refer to a soft drink as *soda* or *pop*. In northern parts of the United States, *sugar* refers to a sweetener. In the South and Appalachia, *sugar* can also refer to a kiss, as when a grandparent says to a grandchild, "Give me some *sugar*." As another example, the Hispanic English phrase "the coat of my father" rather than "my father's coat" reflects a dialectic variation affecting syntax. In this chapter, we will provide examples and information on both accent and dialect.

DIFFERENT VIEWS OF DIALECT

Two views regarding dialect are commonly found: sociolinguistic and deficit. The sociolinguistic view, advocated by linguists and other professionals who study languages, characterizes dialect as a difference in the way a person speaks, not a disorder. Professional organizations that advocate the sociolinguistic view of dialect include the Linguistic Society of America (LSA) (1996), the American Dialect Society (ADS) (2001), and the National Council of Teachers of English (NCTE) (Farr, 1991). All these organizations stress the legitimacy of ME-alternative dialects and the importance of allowing their use. In addition, the American Speech-Language-Hearing Association (1983) has stated that "no dialectical variety of English is a disorder or a pathological form of speech or language." (p. 78). Thus, a person's language usage that is communicatively appropriate to other speakers in the community but different from another's (noncommunity member) language usage is considered a language difference, not a language deficit or disorder.

Unfortunately for many non-ME speakers, the general public tends to view alternative dialects from a "deficit" viewpoint. From this perspective, dialect is viewed as a deviation from ME. It needs to be changed or even eliminated so that the non-ME speaker "talks like everyone else." As a result, some dialects enjoy a higher regard by much of the American public. Dialects such as NEE and ME may be viewed as "better," with Southern English and **Appalachian English (ApE)** viewed less favorably, for example. Similarly, some accents are viewed as more acceptable than others. There are documented cases of social bias and negative reactions based solely on a person's use of non-ME dialect or accent (Buck, Maynard, Garn-Nunn, & Seyfried, 1996; Terrell & Terrell, 1983).

In reality, everyone speaks with an accent (Cheng, 1999). Furthermore, each accent is viewed as acceptable within a person's speech community. The authors both have Midwestern accents, but one was particularly shaped by her late childhood living in the Chicago suburbs. Her accent actually contrasts in some ways from speakers in southern Illinois (where she later lived as an adult for 6 years). As a northern

Illinoisian, she pronounced *Illinois* as [ɪ l ɪ n ɔɪ]. Her elementary school students in the southern part of the state pronounced the state name as [ɪ l ɪ n ɔɪ z]. She also notes speakers who talk about [s t ɑ r m z] coming in from the [n ɑ r θ w ɛ s t] (using [ɑ] for [ɔ]). For her, that particular pronunciation is associated with St. Louis and southeast Missouri speakers, again discovered while she lived and worked in southern Illinois.

Dialect and accent use also compose an important part of "belonging" in a particular social group or community. As Cheng (1999, p. 1) has noted:

> Everyone speaks with an accent. This accent tells his/her life story, where he/she has been, where he/she is from, where he/she learned his/her language, what cultures he/she has been exposed to. In sum, it is the way to tell the world who he/she is. To take this away is to take a part of his/her history away.

It might surprise you to know that attitudes about dialects vary among different speakers and language communities. A Southern English speaker might be viewed as "slow" by an ME speaker, but the ME speaker may be regarded as "snobbish" by a community of SE speakers. Sometimes, alternative dialect speakers find it necessary to "code switch." Appalachian English–speaking students of the first author often used a different dialect at college (more ME-sounding) but continued to use Appalachian English in their home environment. As they explained it, community (college or home) acceptance required that they speak that community's dialect. Other students continued to use Appalachian English in all settings. They felt that the dialect expressed who they were and that people should have to accept them that way.

As we noted earlier, most professional organizations view dialects as different but equally valid ways to communicate. Speech-language pathologists who work with dialect speakers do not do so because their speech is disordered. Instead, they help their clients to sound more mainstream in certain situations while valuing the original dialect in appropriate settings. The idea is to expand dialect capacities rather than stamp out any evidence of the non-ME dialect.

SOURCES OF DIALECTIC VARIATION

REGIONAL DIALECTS

Regional dialects are those characteristic of speakers in certain regions of the United States. We have already mentioned several regional dialects, SE, NEE, and ApE. These dialects evolved for a variety of reasons, including settlers' area of origin and possible geographic isolation in their new homes. Table 8–1 depicts common U.S. regional dialects and where they are found. Note that this is not an all-inclusive list. Smaller dialect areas can (and do) exist within these regions. Additionally, the number and boundaries of the regions identified can vary somewhat, depending on the researcher and date of study (Kurath & McDavid, 1961; Labov, 1991, 1997).

Table 8–2 contrasts ME characteristics with those of NE, SE, and ApE. Notice that these dialects are much more like ME than they are different from it. You will also find some surprising similarities among these variants of ME (e.g., SE and NE).

TABLE 8–1 SOME U.S. REGIONAL DIALECTS AND THEIR AREAS OF USAGE

Dialect	Abbreviation	Geographic Areas of Usage
New England	NEE	ME, NH, RI; eastern portions of MA, VT
Appalachian English	ApE	WV, western MD, PA, VA, NC; eastern KY, TN
Southern American English	SAE/SE	Coastal and eastern VA; NC, SC, GA, FL, AL, MS, LA; southern OK; central and eastern TX
Great Lakes English	GLE	Northern PA; central and western NY; northern OH, IN, IL; lower MI, southeastern WI
North Central English	NCE	MI, MN, WI; middle and eastern ND, SD; MI Upper Peninsula
Central Midland	CME	MO, central IL, northern OK (including panhandle); KS, NB, CO, western TX; southeastern WY
Northwest English	NWE	ID, MT, WY, WA, OR, northern CA, NV, UT
Southwest English	SWE	AZ; central and southern NV, central and southern CA

Sources: McLaughlin (1998); Salvucci (1999).

TABLE 8–2 COMPARISON OF SELECTED CHARACTERISTICS OF REGIONAL DIALECTS IN U.S.A.

Mainstream	New England	Southern	Appalachian
Postvocalic / ɹ /:	Elongated/Diphthongized		
[k a ɹ]	[k a :]	[k a :]	Same as ME
[f ɔ ɹ]	[f o ə]	[f o:]	Same as ME
Vowels			
[ɝ ɚ]:			
[w ɝ]	[w ɜ]	Same as NEE	Same as ME
[h æ m ɚ]	[h æ m ə]	Same as NEE	Same as ME
/æ/	broad *a*/NE *a*	Same as ME	Same as ME
[æ sk]	[a s k]		
[b a θ]	[b a θ]		
/aɪ/			
[h aɪ]	Same as ME	[h ɑ:]	Same as SE
[n aɪ s]	Same as ME	[n ɑ s]	Same as SE
/ɪ/–/ɛ/ (before nasal)			
[p ɪ n] (pin)	Same as ME	Same as ME	Same as ME
[p ɛ n] (pen)	Same as ME	[p ɪ n]	Same as SE
/ə/ in unstressed syllables			
[s æ l ə d] (salad)	Same as ME	[s æ l ɪ d]	Same as SE
[l ɛ t ə s] (lettuce)	Same as ME	[l ɛ t ɪs]	Same as SE
[b ə l i v] (believe)	Same as ME	[b ɪ l i v]	Same as SE
/u/ in selected words			
[studənt] (student)	[s t j u d ə n t]	Same as NEE	Same as ME
[t u n] (tune)	[t j u n]	Same as NEE	Same as ME

Sources: Calvert (1992); Salvucci (1999); Wolfram (1991).

Cultural/Ethnic Dialects

Another source of dialectic variation in the United States is associated with different cultures or ethnic backgrounds. The accent of a speaker of Asian-American English, for example, might differ from mainstream English in certain characteristics. The extent of such differences will depend on a number of factors, including original or first language used, language(s) spoken in the home, and schooling. We will discuss three cultural dialects in this section: African-American English (AAE), Hispanic English (HE), and Asian English (AE). Take note: Individuals from one of these cultures may not necessarily use the dialect characteristics. Use can vary according to family customs, conversational partners, and situational factors. We previously noted that speakers of regional dialects may shift their dialect usage, depending on the situation and listeners. The same principle also holds true for speakers of AAE, HE, and AE. In addition, the regional dialect will affect any cultural dialect used. Consequently, an AE speaker living in the South will not sound exactly like an AE speaker who lives in Minnesota. Nevertheless, there are certain characteristics for each of these dialects that have been identified as occurring more frequently among speakers. We will discuss these in this part of the chapter.

African-American English (AAE)

Other terms used for this dialect include **African-American vernacular English (AAVE),** Black English, and Ebonics. In each case, the term refers to a dialect of English that shares characteristics common to the languages of West Africa (vanKeulen, Weddington, & DeBose, 1998) and Southern American English (Wolfram, 1994). An individual's use of AAE will depend on several factors, particularly listener identity and situational contexts. Like speakers of some regional dialects, AAE speakers can find it necessary to be "bidialectical" (vanKeulen et al., 1998). The ethnic background of African Americans' listeners and the degree of formality of a speaking situation will affect AAE use. AAE differs somewhat from ME in certain aspects of phonology, morphology, and syntax. Tables 8–3, 8–4, and 8–5 show the pronunciation characteristics most often cited for AAE.

Hispanic English

Americans of Hispanic origin are expected to be the largest minority group in the United States by 2020 (Perez, 1994). Consequently, the number of individiuals who use this dialect continues to grow. Just because someone is of Hispanic origin or uses HE does not mean that all HE speakers will sound alike. Factors affecting HE use include the speaker's country of origin and the type of Spanish spoken. Not all HE speakers come from the same country, of course. Immigrants and first-generation Americans of Spanish origins could be from Cuba, Puerto Rico, Central America, or South America, as well as from Spain and other countries. There are also different types of Spanish, just as there are dialects in English. Depending on the person's original Spanish use, HE use can vary. Usage can also differ according to the language (Spanish or English) spoken in the home and by extended family and friends. Some speakers will be fully bilingual; others will not. The degree of English proficiency can vary according to all these factors plus the amount of time spent in the United States and the nature of the speaker's schooling. And, like AE

TABLE 8–3 FREQUENTLY CITED PRONUNCIATION CHARACTERISTICS OF AAE:
SINGLETON CONSONANTS

Consonant Singletons	Prevocalic	AAE Usage Intervocalic	Postvocalic
Nasals: /m/ /n/			May be omitted with nasalization of the preceding vowel
Nasal /ŋ/			/n/ for unstressed -ing
Stops			May be omitted
Voiced fricatives /v/ /z/ / /			May be omitted
/θ/		/f/	/f/
/ð/	/d/	/d/	/d/ or /v/
/r/			Omitted or /ə/

Sources: Kamhi, Pollack, & Harris (1996); Williams & Wolfram, (1977); Wolfram (1994).

TABLE 8–4 FREQUENTLY CITED CHARACTERISTICS OF AAE: CONSONANT SEQUENCES

	AAE Usage	Example
Prevocalic		
/θr/	/θ/	throw [θ oʊ]
/ʃr/	/sr/	shrimp [s r ɪmp]
/s t r]	/s k r]	street [s k r i t]
Postvocalic		
/l/ + nasal	/l/ omitted	helm [hɛm]
		kiln [kɪn]
/l/ + stop	/l/ omitted	help [hɛp]
		melt [mɛt]
		milk [mɪk]
/l/ + fricative	/l/ omitted	self [sɛf]
Nasal + stop	Stop omitted	dump [dʌm]
		dent [dɛn]
		hand [h æ n]
		drink [dr ɪ n]
Fricative + /p/, /t/	Stop omitted	crisp [kr ɪs]
		last [l æ s]
		coughed [kɔf]
/k/ + /s/	Segments reversed	ask [ae ks]
3-element sequences	Variable phoneme omission	length [l ɛŋkθ] [l ɛn f]
		sinks [s ɪ ŋ ks] [sɪns]
		text [t ɛ k s]

Sources: Kamhi, Pollack, & Harris (1996); Williams & Wolfram (1977); Wolfram (1994).

TABLE 8–5 FREQUENTLY CITED CHARACTERISTICS OF AAE VOWELS AND DIPHTHONGS

Vowel	AAE Usage	Example
/ɛ/	Shift to /ɪ/ before nasals	Ben [bɪn]
		hem [hɪm]
/ɝ/	/ɜ/	turn [tɜn]
/ɚ/	/ə/	under [ʌndə]
/aɪ/	/ɑ/	eyes [ɑz]
/ɔɪ/	/ɔ/	boil [bɔl]

Sources: Kamhi, Pollack, & Harris (1996); Williams & Wolfram (1977); Wolfram (1994).

speakers, HE speakers' characteristics will also show some variation according to geographic region in the United States. Despite these factors, a core of phonological characteristics has been identified as most typical of HE speakers. These are displayed in Tables 8–6 and 8–7. Some of these characteristics are easier to understand if you know something about Spanish. First, Spanish has fewer vowels than English. Consequently, substitutions of similar vowels can result. Note in Table 8–6

TABLE 8–6 FREQUENTLY CITED CHARACTERISTICS OF HE VOWELS AND DIPHTHONGS

Vowel/Diphthong	HE Usage	Examples
/i/	/ɪ/	eat [ɪ t]
		seat [s ɪ t]
/ɪ/	/i/	sit [s i t]
		is [i z]
/ɛ/	/æ/	bed [b æ d]
		said [s æ d]
	/eɪ/	said [s eɪ d]
/æ/	/ɛ/	bat [b ɛ t]
		Sam [s ɛ m]
/u/	/ʊ/	news [n ʊ z]
		soon [s ʊ n]
/ʊ/	/u/	book [b u k]
		hood [h u d]
/ɔ/	/oʊ/	hall [h oʊ l]
		tall [t oʊ l]
/ʌ/	/ɑ/	duck [d ɑ k]
		puppy [p ɑ p i]
/ɝ/	/ɛɹ/	her [h ɛɹ]
		purr [p ɛɹ]

Sources: Owens RE (1992); Perez (1994).

TABLE 8–7 FREQUENTLY CITED CHARACTERISTICS OF HE CONSONANTS

Consonant Singleton	HE Usage		
	Initial	Medial	Final
Stops			
/p t/			Omitted/distorted
/b k g/			Omitted/distorted/cognate
/d/		Dentalized	
Fricatives			
/f/			Omitted
/v/	/b/	/b/	Distorted
/θ/	/t/ /s/	Omitted	/t/ /s/
/ð/	/d/	/d/ /z/ /v/	/d/
/z/	/s/	/s/	/s/
/ʃ/	/tʃ/	/s/ /tʃ/	/tʃ/
Affricates			
/tʃ/	/ʃ/	/ʃ/	/ʃ/
/dʒ/	/d/	/j/	/ʃ/
Nasals			
/m/			Omitted
/ŋ/		/d/	/n/
Liquids and Glides			
/w/	/hu/		
/j/	/dʒ/		
/ɹ/	Distorted	Distorted	Distorted
Consonant Sequences			
/s/ = sequences	/ɛ/ + sequence		

Source: Owens (1992); Perez (1994).

how both /i/ and /ɪ/ may be interchanged. Spanish phonology includes /i/ but not /ɪ/, which explains how the two phonemes may be used variably in English. In addition to the variations noted in Table 8–6, HE speakers may substitute monophthong /e/ and /o/ for the diphthongs /eɪ/ and /oʊ/, respectively.

Some ME-HE consonant differences result from Spanish consonant phonemes being substituted for English phonemes. Other substitutions result because an English phoneme is absent in Spanish. In particular, substitutions will be found for /v z θ ʒ/. Also, alveolar stops and nasal /n/ may be dentalized in HE, as they are in Spanish. Other commonly observed HE characteristics include deletion of most final consonants because very few consonants (only /s n ɹ l d/) occur in the final word position in Spanish (Perez, 1994). See Table 8–7 for additional consonant characteristics.

ASIAN-PACIFIC ISLANDER (API)/ASIAN ENGLISH (AE)

Americans who trace their origins from Asian countries and the Pacific Islands constitute another fast-growing ethnic group within the United States. Like any other minority dialect group, API Americans may experience communication interference and discrimination, based on their dialect. The term *Asian English* is actually misleading, making it sound as though one, uniform dialect characterizes the speech of all Americans of API origin. As with other ethnic dialects, a variety of factors can affect use of AE.

First, Americans of Asian extraction come from a variety of countries and represent a large number of native languages. A speaker of AE could come from China, Japan, Southeast Asia, India, or any one of a number of different Pacific Islands. But even AE speakers coming from the same country will not necessarily share all their dialect characteristics. AE speakers from China may speak Cantonese, or they may use Mandarin. These languages differ from each other and from English in the number of consonants and vowels, as well as in permissible phoneme arrangements. Both languages differ from English in being tonal languages in which intonation actually signals a change in meaning. A particular CVC can vary in meaning in Mandarin depending on which tonal pattern is used to produce it; for example, upper even or lower even (Cheng, 1994). Nevertheless, Mandarin and Cantonese still differ from each other in the number of tones used to signal meaning. Thus, actual AE characteristics will depend heavily on the speaker's native language and any other languages that might have affected the native language.

Other influences on AE are similar to those affecting speakers of other ethnic dialects. Is the speaker newly arrived to the United States or a longtime resident? First or second generation in this country? What dialect of English did he or she originally learn? (Immigrants from India, for example, will use British English additionally influenced by their native languages, which might be Hindi, Punjabi, or Bengali.) At what age was English learned? Which language is used at home and at school? All these factors and more can affect AE speaker characteristics.

After reading the previous paragraphs, you may understand why we are somewhat reluctant to list typical characteristics of AE as we have done for AAE and HE. Nevertheless, we can make some generalizations about probable characteristics used by AE speakers. Vowel confusions may be expected, often involving /ɪ/ (varying with /i/) and /æ/ (replaced by /e/) (Cheng, 1994). Other vowels that may be produced differently include /ɔ/ and /ʊ/. Final consonant omission may be found in AE speakers because their native languages have few, if any, final consonants. Consonant clusters or sequences may also be particularly difficult or affected by epenthesis (addition of a sound, usually /ə/, e.g., *black* [bə l æ k]. Again, consonant sequences do not occur in all Asian languages, which can strongly affect AE usage (Cheng, 1994; Iglesias & Goldstein, 1998).

Several consonants are more prone than others to change, especially liquid /ɹ/ and the voiceless and voiced interdental fricatives /θ/ and /ð/. The liquids /l/ and /ɹ/ are frequently confused in AE, particularly in the prevocalic and intervocalic positions. Also, s/θ, f/θ, and d/ð substitutions frequently occur in AE.

Everyone in the United States speaks a dialect. Some are more widely used than others, but all are equally valid language systems. Dialects emerge because of a variety of factors, including region of settlement, possible geographic isolation, and country of national origin. Despite the validity of different dialects, society tends to place value judgments on them, viewing some dialects as "better" than others. For speakers who find that their dialect creates communication difficulties, accent reduction/expansion programs are available. Discussion of these and other uses of applied phonetics will be found in Chapter 9.

REVIEW VOCABULARY

accent   phonological and suprasegmental characteristics of dialect.

African-American vernacular English (AAVE)   cultural dialect used by many, but not all, African Americans.

Appalachian English (ApE)   regional dialect used by speakers in the Appalachian region of the United States.

cultural dialect   dialect associated with a particular cultural group (e.g., AAVE).

dialect   set of phonological, morphological, and syntactic characteristics that characterize a particular way of speaking American English.

ebonics   see AAVE.

English as a second language (ESL) speaker: individual who learned (an)other language(s) prior to learning English.

mainstream (American) English (ME)   form of American English most commonly used in textbooks and in national broadcast media; also known as general American English.

New England (American) English (NEE)   regional dialect used by speakers in the northeastern United States.

regional dialect   dialect associated with a particular geographic region of the United States.

southern (American) English (SE)   regional dialect used by speakers in the Deep South of the United States.

standard American English (SAE)   American English dialect characteristic of education and textbooks; also known as general or mainstream American English.

EXERCISES

1. Say the following words to yourself, then transcribe them. Next, find someone whose accent seems different from yours and ask him or her to say these words. Transcribe their productions. Are there any differences? What are your dialect backgrounds?

    a. cot   [   ] [   ] caught [   ] [   ]
    b. not   [   ] [   ] naught [   ] [   ]
    c. Ott   [   ] [   ] ought   [   ] [   ]
    d. all   [   ] [   ] oil   [   ] [   ]
    e. pin   [   ] [   ] pen   [   ] [   ]
    f. windy   [   ] [   ] Wendy   [   ] [   ]
    g. bit   [   ] [   ] beet   [   ] [   ]
    h. cud   [   ] [   ] could   [   ] [   ]

i.   higher   [   ]   [   ]
j.   faster   [   ]   [   ]

2. *Regional dialects:* For the following, indicate the most likely regional dialect of the speaker (e.g., NEE, SE, ApE).

	Examples	**Probable Regional Dialect**
a.	mine→[m ɑ n]	
	hide→[h ɑ d]	
b.	bird→[b ɜ d]	
	ladder→[læ d ə]	
c.	handed→[h æ n d ɪ d]	
	palace→[p æ l ɪ s]	
d.	sent→[s ɛ n t]	
	lend→[l ɛ n d]	

3. African-American English (AAE): using Tables 8–3, 8–4, and 8–5, transcribe the following words as they might be said in AAE.

a.	**meant**	[ ]	e.	**burst**	[ ]
b.	**fine**	[ ]	f.	**shelf**	[ ]
c.	**other**	[ ]	g.	**birth**day	[ ]
d.	**herself**	[ ]	h.	**desk**	[ ]

4. *Hispanic English:* Using Tables 8–6 and 8–7, transcribe the following words as they might be produced in HE.

a.	**very**	[ ]	e.	**skirt**	[ ]
	shovel	[ ]		**scurry**	[ ]
b.	**breathe**	[ ]	f.	**call**	[ ]
	teeth	[ ]		**law**	[ ]
c.	**choose**	[ ]	g.	**ship**	[ ]
	juice	[ ]		**chip**	[ ]
d.	**which**	[ ]	h.	**thumb**	[ ]
	win	[ ]		**sung**	[ ]

CHAPTER 9

APPLIED PHONETICS

ARTICULATORY AND PHONOLOGIC DISORDERS
ENGLISH AS A SECOND LANGUAGE (ESL)
VOICE AND DICTION TRAINING
REVIEW VOCABULARY
EXERCISES

So far this book has been devoted to developing basic and advanced skills in the transcription of American English with its dialectic variations. There are additional uses for phonetics beyond transcription of normal speech, however. Knowledge and application of phonetics are instrumental to the work of linguists, speech-language pathologists, audiologists, ESL instructors, and speech trainers/coaches, to mention just a few professionals who use applied phonetics in their work. This chapter will discuss some of the applications of phonetics in different professions.

ARTICULATORY AND PHONOLOGIC DISORDERS

Traditionally, speech-language pathologists, who work with clients who have articulatory and phonologic disorders, require a thorough knowledge of phonetics and phonology. People with **articulation disorders** have difficulty in producing the sounds of their native language. In **phonologic disorders** (most often occurring in children), there is a failure to master the sound system of the language. The effects on speech of such disorders can range from a simple lisp (/s/ problem) to the loss of whole sound classes, for example, deletion of final consonants, **stopping** (replacing fricatives with stops), and **velar fronting** (alveolar phonemes replace velar phonemes). In order to treat such problems, speech-language pathologists must be able to transcribe the client's speech, determine errors, and explain the placement and manner of phoneme formation to the client as part of treatment.

ASSESSMENT IN ARTICULATORY AND PHONOLOGIC DISORDERS

Before setting treatment goals for clients with articulatory and phonologic disorders, the speech-language pathologist must collect a representative sample of a particular client's speech. There are a number of ways to collect speech samples for analysis. Most often, speech-language pathologists use some type of speech sound inventory or formal test in evaluation. The client is asked to name pictures or to read words or sentences. Any errors are transcribed phonetically. Some tests evaluate mastery of phonemes (phonemic tests), whereas others are designed to examine the client's understanding of phonological rules (phonology tests). A conversational sample should also be collected and analyzed.

Phonemic or "one sound at a time" tests typically test every English consonant in three consonant **word positions, initial**/prevocalic, **medial**/intervocalic, and **final**/postvocalic. Such tests may or may not include words for evaluating vowel accuracy. Most often, errors are classified in one of four ways: omission, substitution, distortion, or addition. In a phoneme **omission,** the client deletes or omits the tested phoneme; for example, *bicycle* is produced as [b aɪ ɪ k ə l] (/s/ omitted in the medial/intervocalic position). When one standard speech sound replaces another standard speech sound, a **substitution** has occurred; for example, *bicycle* is produced as [b aɪ θɪ k ə l], a substitution of θ/s in the medial position. A **distortion** occurs when a standard speech sound is replaced by a nonstandard speech sound. Often, transcription of distortions requires the use of narrow transcription. Finally, a sound is added to a word in an **addition;** for example, *bicycle* might be produced as [b aɪ sɪ k ə l i] for an addition in the final or postvocalic position. Table 9–1 gives examples of scoring for a phonemic test.

Phonology tests require whole word transcription or recording of every error made. Each production is then examined for phonological rules used by the client. Some tests also allow for assessment of both phoneme and phonological rule mastery. In all cases, the collection of a speech sample requires the phonetic transcription of a client's speech. The speech-language pathologist must then analyze the errors to determine if a problem exists and the probable goals of treatment.

TABLE 9–1   EXAMPLES OF SCORING FOR A PHONEMIC TEST

Test Phoneme/ Position (I, M, F)	Stimulus Word	Response	Error Recording
/s/ (I)	sun	[θʌn]	θ/s (I)
(M)	bicycle	[baɪθɪkəl]	θ/s (M)
(F)	house	[haʊ]	-/s (F)
/ʃ/ (I)	shoe	[su]	s/ʃ (I)
(M)	dishes	[dɪsəz]	s/ʃ (M)
(F)	fish	[fɪtʃ]	tʃ/ʃ (F)
/l/ (I)	lamp	[wæmp]	w/l (I)
(M)	balloon	[bəwun]	w/l (M)
(F)	bell	[bɛ]	-/l (F)
/ɹ/ (I)	red	[wɛd]	w/ɹ (I)
(M)	carry	[kɛwi]	w/ɹ (M)
(F)	door	[dɔə]	ə/ɹ (F)

Note. / indicates "in place of"; - indicates omission.
F = final/postvocalic
I = initial/prevocalic
M = medial/intervocalic

TABLE 9–2 SCORING FOR USE OF PHONOLOGICAL PROCESSES

Target Word	Transcription	Processes Used					
		Syllable Deletion	Final Consonant Deletion	Stopping	Velar Fronting	Gliding	Vowelization
sun	[t ʌ]		✓	✓			
bicycle	[tɪzko]	✓	✓	✓			✓
house	[h aʊ]		✓	✓			
shoe	[t u]			✓			
dishes	[d ɪ t ə]		✓	✓			
fish	[p ɪ]		✓	✓			
light	[w aɪ]		✓				
balloon	[b u]	✓	✓				
bell	[b ɛ o]					✓	✓
red	[w ɛ]		✓				
carry	[t ɛ w i]				✓	✓	
door	[d ɔ]		✓				

ANALYSIS OF ARTICULATORY AND PHONOLOGIC ERRORS

Transcribed results from phonemic tests may be analyzed in several ways. The most commonly used procedure is to determine the specific sounds that are in error and in what position(s) these errors occur. Further error analysis may include classifying errors according to place, manner, and voicing confusions.

For the results from phonology tests, the speech-language pathologist looks for the use of rules or processes to account for the errors noted in the client's speech. A child who consistently omitted the final consonant in the words tested would be considered to have a problem with **final consonant deletion.** Velar fronting is the process used to describe the following error pattern in which alveolar consonants replace all velar consonants: t/k, d/g, and n/ŋ. Substitutions of p/f, b/v, t/θ, t/s, d/z, t/ʃ, and d/ʒ, which involve seven different phonemes, all represent one rule of misunderstanding: stopping. In stopping, stops replace fricatives. (See Table 9–2 for an example of an abbreviated phonological process analysis of a child's responses.)

INTERPRETATION OF RESULTS

How do we decide whether misarticulations or use of **phonological processes** actually indicate that our client has a problem? We turn to age norms, either included as part of a standardized test or developed from research (Arlt & Goodban, 1976; Prather, Hedrick, & Kern, 1975; Sander, 1972; Smit, Hand, Freilinger, Bernthal, & Bird, 1990; Templin, 1957). If a client is using phonological processes that should have been eliminated by his or her chronological age, a phonological disorder is indicated. Similarly, phoneme mastery norms indicate that all American phonemes should be acquired by age 8. Consequently, misarticulation of /s/ or /ʧ/ should not occur after that age. (See Table 9–3 for examples of ages of phoneme mastery and Table 9–4 for ages of phonological process dissolution.)

TABLE 9–3 SAMPLE AGES (IN YEARS) OF MASTERY FOR SELECTED PHONEMES

Phoneme	Sander (1972)[1]	Prather, Hedrick, and Kern (1975)	Smit et al. (1990)[2]
/p/	3	2	3
/k/	4	2–4	3
/s/	8	3	9
/θ/	7	4	6
/m/	3	2	3
/n/	3	2	3–6
/ɹ/	6	3–4	8
/j/	3	2–4	4
/l/	6	2–8	6

[1]Based on data collected by Templin (1957) and Wellman, Case, Mengert, and Bradbury (1931). Number indicates age of mastery (sound produced correctly by 90% of children tested). Other researchers have used different criteria to indicate mastery.

[2]Based on a normative study of children in Iowa and Nebraska, with testing in initial and final positions only. Ages reported are those for girls; up to age 7, there were sometimes small differences between the ages of acquisition for males and females.

TABLE 9–4 AGES OF LOSS OF SELECTED PHONOLOGICAL PROCESSES

Process	Chronological Age (in years)
Unstressed syllable deletion	≤ 4
Final consonant deletion	≤ 3–6
Velar fronting	≤ 3–6
Gliding	≥ 4
Vowelization	≥ 4

Note. Ages are based on the following studies: Grunwell (1982); Haelsig and Madison (1986); Hodson and Paden (1981); Lowe, Knutson, and Monson (1985).

Speech-language pathologists also consider speech intelligibility level as well as several other factors in deciding if the client has a problem. If an articulation problem exists, the speech-language pathologist designs a treatment program to help the client develop the phoneme or phonemes in error. For the child with a phonological problem, a treatment program can be designed to help the child develop age-appropriate rule use. For example, we might teach the child to "close/finish the word" (final consonant deletion) or contrast "front tongue" and "back tongue" sounds (velar fronting).

Once error analysis has been completed, the speech-language pathologist can set goals and begin actual treatment. The type and frequency of treatment will depend on a number of factors, including the nature and severity of the articulation or phonologic disorder.

ENGLISH AS A SECOND LANGUAGE (ESL)

To qualify as a TESOL (Teaching English to Speakers of Other Languages) instructor, you must take specific college course work and meet certification requirements. Training in phonetics is included as part of the curriculum, along with study in linguistics, sociolinguistics, grammar, and syntax. Course work in testing and teaching reading, writing, and speaking skills of students is also part of the course of study. TESOL instructors may work in a variety of settings, including public schools, colleges and universities, and agencies that serve immigrants to the United States.

VOICE AND DICTION TRAINING

A number of professionals may be involved with helping individuals improve the clarity and effectiveness of their speech. These include speech-language pathologists and coaches or teachers of voice and diction. Clients for these services may include business people and other professionals who wish to improve their communication effectiveness. Actors and actresses who need to use an alternative dialect for a dramatic role may also seek the services of such a coach. Because pronunciation is targeted, a knowledge of phonetics is crucial for a diction coach or teacher. Knowledge of how phonemes are made and the ability to transcribe using the IPA system are very important to success in such training.

REVIEW VOCABULARY

addition   articulation error in which a phoneme is added to a word.

articulation disorder   consistent misarticulation of a phoneme or phonemes; related to motoric difficulty in forming speech sounds.

distortion   phoneme error in which a nonstandard sound replaces a standard speech sound.

final consonant deletion   phonological process in which the child or adult omits consonants at the end of words.

gliding   phonological process affecting liquids; the glide /w/ or /j/ replaces /l/ and/or /ɹ/.

initial, medial, final   traditional terms referring to the position of a phoneme in a word; pre, inter, and postvocalic.

omission   phoneme error in which the child or adult deletes a phoneme regardless of position.

phonologic(al) disorder   failure to master the sound system of a language.

phonological process   error pattern affecting a particular class of phonemes; see Final Consonant Deletion, Stopping, Velar Fronting.

stopping   phonological process in which stops are substituted for fricatives; for example, *soap* is produced as [t oʊp].

substitution   phoneme error in which one standard speech sound replaces another standard speech sound.

velar fronting   phonological process in which velars (k g ŋ] are replaced by more anterior consonants, for example, t/k, d/g, n/ŋ.

vowelization   phonological process affecting postvocalic liquids; a vowel replaces postvocalic /ɹ/ or /l/ (e.g., *bell* is produced as [b ɛ o]). May also be referred to as vocalization.

word position   traditional articulation test term, referring to the place of a particular phoneme in a word: see Initial, Medial, Final.

EXERCISES

1. For the following speech sample, transcribe the error and indicate the position in which it occurs. The first two examples have been completed for you.

Test Phoneme	Stimulus Word	Client's Production	Error/ Position(s)
/k/	cup	[tʌp]	
	rocket	[rɑtɪt]	
	rake	[reɪt]	
			t/k (I, M, F)

Test Phoneme	Stimulus Word	Client's Production	Error/ Position(s)
/g/	gum	[d ʌ m]	
	wagon	[w æ d ə n]	
	pig	[p ɪ g]	
			d/g (I, M)
/ʧ/	chair	[ʃ ɛ ɹ]	
	matches	[m æ ʧ ɪ z]	
	watch	[w ɑ ʃ]	
/ʒ/	treasure	[t ɹ ɛ ɚ]	
	garage	[g ə ɹ ɑ d]	
/θ/	thumb	[f ʌ m]	
	toothpaste	[t u p eɪ s t]	
	teeth	[t i f]	

2. For the following speech sample, indicate which of the selected phonological processes are used in each word. The two examples have been completed for you.

Target Word	Transcription	Final Consonant Deletion	Stopping	Velar Fronting	Gliding
cup	[tʌ]	X		X	
rocket	[wɑtɪ]	X		X	X
rake	[weɪ[				
gum	[dʌ]				
wagon	[wædə]				
pig	[pɪ]				
sun	[tʌ]				
bicycle	[baɪtɪtəl]				
house	[haʊ]				
shoe	[tu]				

What process occurred most often in this sample?

REFERENCES

American Dialect Society. (2001). *Purposes* [Online]. Available: www.americandialect.org.

American Speech-Language-Hearing Association. (1983, September). Position paper: Social dialects and the implications of the position on social dialects. *ASHA, 25*(9), 23–27.

Arlt, P. B., & Goodban, M. T. (1976). A comparative study of articulation acquisition as based on a study of 240 normals, aged three to six. *Language, Speech, and Hearing Services in Schools, 7,* 173–180.

Buck, S., Maynard, D., Garn-Nunn, P., & Seyfried, D. (1996). Appalachian English speakers and naive listeners: Potential for listener bias and communication interference. *Journal of the Speech-Language-Hearing Association of Virginia, 36,* 24–33.

Calvert, D. (1992). *Descriptive Phonetics* (2nd ed.). New York: Thieme Medical Publishers.

Cheng, L. L. (1994). Asian-Pacific students and the learning of English. In J. E. Bernthal & N. W. Bankson (Eds.), *Child phonology: Characteristics, assessment, and intervention with special populations* (pp. 255–274). New York: Thieme Medical Publishers.

Cheng, L. L. (1999). Moving beyond accent: Social and cultural realities of living with many tongues. *Topics in Language Disorders, 19*(4), 1–10.

Chomsky, N., & Halle, M. (1968). *The sound pattern of English.* New York: Harper & Row.

Cunningham, R. (1993). *Southern talk: A disappearing language.* Asheville, NC: Bright Mountain Books.

Farr, M. (1991). Dialects, culture, and teaching the English language arts. In J. Flood, J. M. Jensen, D. Lap, & J. Squire (Eds.), *Handbook of research on teaching the English language arts.* New York: Macmillan.

Grunwell, P. (1982). *Clinical phonology.* London: Croom Helm.

Haelsig, P. C., & Madison, C. L. (1986). A study of phonological processes exhibited by 3-, 4-, and 5-year-old children. *Language, Speech, and Hearing Services in Schools, 17,* 107–114.

Hodson, B. W., & Paden, E. P. (1981). Phonological processes which characterize unintelligible and intelligible speech in early childhood. *Journal of Speech and Hearing Disorders, 46,* 369–373.

Iglesias, A., & Goldstein, B. (1998). Language and dialectal variations. In J. E. Bernthal & N. W. Bankson (Eds.), *Child phonology: Characteristics, assessment, and intervention with special populations* (pp. 148–171). New York: Thieme Medical Publishers.

International Phonetic Association (2002). *The International Phonetic Association.* [Online]: Available: www.arts.gla.ac.uk/IPA/ipa.html.

Kamhi, A. G., Pollack, K.E., & Harris, J. L. (1996). *Communication development and disorders in African American children.* Baltimore: Paul H. Brookes.

Kurath, H., & McDavid, R. I. (1961). *The pronunciation of English in the Atlantic States, based upon the collections of the linguistic atlas of the Eastern United States.* Ann Arbor: University of Michigan Press.

Labov, W. (1991). The three dialects of English. In P. Eckert (Ed.), *New ways of analyzing sound change* (pp. 1–44). San Diego, CA: Academic Press.

Labov, W. (1997). Linguistics and sociolinguistics. In N. Coupland & A. Jaworkski (Eds.), *Sociolinguistics: A reader* (pp. 23–24). New York: St. Martin's Press.

Linguistic Society of America. (1996, update 1998). Statement on language rights [Online]. Available: www.lsadc.org/web2/resolutionsfr.html.

Lowe, R. J., Knutson, P. J., & Monson, M. A. (1985). Incidence of fronting in preschool children. *Language, Speech, and Hearing Services in Schools, 16,* 119–123.

McLaughlin, S. (1998). *Introduction to language development.* San Diego, CA: Singular Publishing Group.

Montgomery, J. (1999). Accents and dialects: Creating a national professional statement. *Topics in Language Disorders, 19*(4), 78–88.

National Council of Teachers of English. (2001). Position statements. [Online]. Available: www.ncte.org/positions.

Ohde, R., & Sharf, D. (1992). *Phonetic analysis of normal and abnormal speech.* New York: Merrill.

Owens, R. E. (1992). *Language development: An introduction* (3rd ed.). New York: Merrill.

Perez, E. (1994). Phonological differences among speakers of Spanish-influenced English. In J. E. Bernthal & N. W. Bankson (Eds.), *Child phonology: Characteristics, assessment, and intervention with special populations* (pp. 245–254). New York: Thieme Medical Publishers.

Prather, E., Hedrick, D., & Kern, C. (1975). Articulation development in children aged two to four years. *Journal of Speech and Hearing Research, 40,* 55–63.

Salvucci, C. (1999). The American Dialect Homepage [Online]: Available: www.evolpub.com/Americandialects.

Sander, E. (1972). When are speech sounds learned? *Journal of Speech and Hearing Disorders, 37,* 55–63.

Shriberg, L., & Kent, R. (1982). *Clinical phonetics.* New York: John Wiley & Sons.

Shriberg, L., & Kent, R. (1995). *Clinical phonetics.* Boston: Allyn & Bacon.

Smit, A. B., Hand, L., Freilinger, J. J., Bernthal, J. E., & Bird, A. (1990). The Iowa Articulation Norms and its Nebraska replication. *Journal of Speech and Hearing Disorders, 55,* 779–798.

Templin, M. C. (1957). *Certain language skills in children: Their development and interrelationships* (Institute of Child Welfare, Monograph 26). Minneapolis: University of Minnesota Press.

Terrell, S., & Terrell, F. (1983). Effects of speaking Black English on employment opportunities. *ASHA, 25,* 27–29.

vanKeulen, J. E., Weddington, G. T., & DeBose, C. E. (1998). *Speech, language, learning, and the African American child.* Boston: Allyn & Bacon.

Wellman, B., Case, I., Mengert, I., & Bradbury, D. (1931). *Speech sounds of young children*. (University of Iowa Studies in Child Welfare, Monograph 5). Iowa City: University of Iowa Press.

Williams, R. L., & Wolfram, W. (1977). *Social dialects: Differences vs. disorders*. Rockville, MD: American Speech-Language-Hearing Association.

Wolfram, W. (1991). *Dialects and American English*. Englewood Cliffs, NJ: Prentice-Hall.

Wolfram, W. (1994). The phonology of a sociocultural society: The case of African American vernacular English. In J. E. Bernthal & N. W. Bankson (Eds.), *Child phonology: Characteristics, assessment, and intervention with special populations* (pp. 227–244). New York: Thieme Medical Publishers.

Wolfram, W., & Christian, D. (1989). *Dialects and education: Issues and answers*. Englewood Cliffs, NJ: Prentice-Hall.

Wolfram, W., & Fasold, R. W. (1974). *The study of social dialects in American English*. Englewood Cliffs: Prentice-Hall.

ANSWERS TO CHAPTER EXERCISES

CHAPTER 1

CONSONANT EXERCISES

1. (th)orn   fre(sh)   fa(th)er   le(dg)e   (ch)ain   lo(ng)
   wi(sh)   (ph)ony   (th)ink   ri(ng)   wrea(th)   (th)en

2. su(pp)er   pa(ss)ing   pe(tt)ing   lo(tt)o   be(rr)y   wi(ll)ing
   shru(gg)ed   ma(ll)   tri(pp)ed   scu(ff)

3. lim(b)   (k)now   (m)nemonic   (p)sychiatry   (g)nash
   (k)new   (p)salm   paradi(g)m   autum(n)

4. a. chorus   chic
   b. treasure   lose

5. a. zinc   tans   Susan   fuzzy   /z/
   b. mission oceanic sheep   tissue   /ʃ/
   c. singe   jump   badge   gyp   /ʤ/
   d. box   sounds   pace   mercy   /s/
   e. yes   fuse   canyon   onion   /j/
   f. whose   hang   behind   hole   /h/
   g. rough   funny   phoneme graph   /f/
   h. grow   again   begin   pig   /g/

VOWEL EXERCISES

6. b(oa)t   (ou)ter   c(ou)pe   m(ai)d   b(oa)st   r(ou)nd
   m(oo)n   (oi)led   p(ai)n   divi(si)on   s(oo)ner   b(ai)t

7. lod(e)   cag(e)d   enter(e)d   cav(e)   match(e)d   don(e)

8. a. hollow   crow
   b. shoe

9. a. train   feign   lane   paper   /ɑ/
   b. beak   seat   peas   meet   /i/
   c. graph   vat   manic   trash   /æ/
   d. soup   flew   ruse   plume   /u/

e.	possible	palm	bond	soggy	/ɑ/
f.	pun	son	under	trouble	/ʌ/
g.	insist	bitters	pitch	inside	/ɪ/
h.	good	should	cook	full	/ʊ/

CHAPTER 2

1. *Structures associated with terms:*

   a. lips (both)
   b. glottis
   c. teeth
   d. soft palate/velum
   e. pharynx/pharyngeal cavity
   f. nose/nasal cavity
   g. alveolar ridge
   h. hard palate

2. *Supralaryngeal structures:* lips, teeth, alveolar ridge, tongue, hard palate, velum, nasal cavity, oral cavity, nasopharynx, oropharynx, laryngopharynx

3. *Sublaryngeal structures:* trachea, lungs, rib cage, diaphragm

4. *Laryngeal structures and function/location:*

   a. hyoid bone
   b. epiglottis
   c. thyroid cartilage
   d. glottis
   e. arytenoid cartilages
   f. cricoid cartilage
   g. vocal folds

5. *Respiratory cycle pathway:*

   Diaphragm contracts, upward and outward rib cage movement due to muscle action → expansion of thoracic cavity

   Lungs expand (elastic properties) → air drawn into lungs

   Oxygen–carbon dioxide exchange in alveoli

   Actions of gravity, elastic properties of cartilage and lung tissue, muscle relaxation → exhalation via vocal tract

6. Frequency: rate of vibration/cycles per second, measured as Hertz and heard as pitch

   Intensity: relative to vocal fold vibration, refers to extent of displacement of folds; heard as loudness

7. See Figure 2–1 on page 12.

CHAPTER 3

1. Back vowels: /u ʊ o ɔ ɑ/
2. Front vowels: /æ ɛ e ɪ i/

3. Central vowels: /ɝ ɚ ʌ ə/

4. Place of articulation:
   a. bilabial   b. velar   c. palatal   d. alveolar

5. Manner of articulation:
   a. fricative   b. stop   c. glide   d. nasal   e. affricate

6. Phonemes classified by distinctive features:
   a. /d θ s ʃ tʃ n/   d. /k j ŋ u a/
   b. /k ʃ ʒ h tʃ r w/ and vowels   e. /k ʃ tʃ w ŋ i u/
   c. /f v s z ʃ tʃ/

CHAPTER 4

1. Vowels in order of tongue elevation (high to low) /i/ /ɪ/ /e/ /ɛ/ /æ/

2. Back vowels in order of tongue elevation (high to low): /u/ /ʊ/ /o/ /ɔ/ /a/

3. High vowels: /i/ /ɪ/ /u/ /ʊ/

4. Mid vowels: /e/ /ɛ/ /ɝ/ /ɚ/ /ʌ/ /ə/ /o/ /ɔ/

5. Low vowels: /æ/ /a/

6. Shared vowel characteristic: lip rounding

7. Vowel quadrilateral:

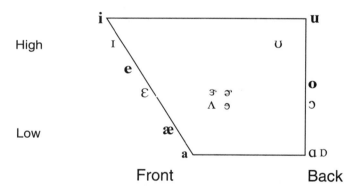

8. I E O A

CHAPTER 5

1. a. /r/ prevocalic singleton   /z/ intervocalic singleton
    b. /b/ prevocalic singleton   /sk/ intervocalic sequence   /t/ postvocalic singleton
    c. /t/ prevocalic singleton   /θ b r/ intervocalic sequence   /ʃ/ postvocalic singleton
    d. /b/ prevocalic singleton   /dh/ intervocalic sequence   /s/ postvocalic sequence
    e. /tʃ/ prevocalic singleton   /r/ postvocalic singleton

f. /l/ prevocalic singleton   /mp/ postvocalic sequence
g. /bl/ prevocalic sequence   /ks/ postvocalic sequence

2. a. /m/   m. /ʒ/
    b. /t/   n. /v/
    c. /ʃ/   o. /b/
    d. /g/   p. /l/
    e. /θ/   q. /p/
    f. /j/   r. /h/
    g. /f/   s. /n/
    h. /tʃ/   t. /d/
    i. /w/   u. /k/
    j. /ð/   v. /ʤ/
    k. /z/   w. /ɹ/
    l. /ŋ/

3. Cognates:
    a. /b/   b. /s/   c. /tʃ/   d. /v/   e. /d/   f. /ʃ/
    g. /ð/   h. /g/

4. Grouped consonants:
    a. /d n z l/
    b. /ʃ ʒ tʃ ʤ j ɹ/
    c. /b d g/
    d. /f θ s ʃ h/
    e. /m n ŋ/
    f. /g ŋ/
    g. /p b m w f v/
    h. /ʤ/

5. Shared characteristics:
    a. Place: alveolar
    b. Place: palatal   Voicing: voiced
    c. Manner: liquids   Voicing: voiced
    d. Place: palatal
    e. Place: velar
    f. Place: alveolar
    g. Voicing: voiced
    h. Place: bilabial

CHAPTER 6

CONNECTED SPEECH

1. Voicing: [̥] [̬]

[θ ɹ̥ i]   [k ɹ̥ u]   [b ɪ h̬ aɪ n d]   [p ɹ̥ eɪ]
[s ɪ t̬ ɪ ŋ] [l ɪ t̬ l̩]   [s l̥ ɪ m]   [θ ɹ̥ ɪ l]
[p l̥ i z]   [f ɹ̥ aɪ]   [ə h̬ ɛ d]   [b ʌ t̬ ɚ]

2. Lengthening: [ː]

[s u n ː oʊ]   [əbaʊtːaɪm]   [b æ d ː eɪ z]
[s ʌ m ː ɛ n]   [b ɪ g ː l æ s]   [r ɪ b ː ʊ nz]
[f ʊ l ː oʊ d]   [b l æ k ː ɑ r]   [r aɪ p ː ɛ r z]
[s p ɛ r ː ɪ b z] [t ɑ p ː ɑ t s]   [ð ɪ s ː ɝ v ə s]

3. Syllabic consonants []

[l ɪ t ḷ]   [r ɪ d n̩]   [b r ɛ d n̩ b ʌ t ɚ]
[k ɪ t n̩]   [b ɑ t ḷ]   [r ɪ d ḷ]
[k æ t ḷ]   [i d n̩]   [k ʌ d ḷ]
[d ɪ g n̩]   [m i t m̩]   [d r ɪ v n̩]

4. Intrusion: [t] [p] [k] [w] [j]

[tʃ æ n t s]   [s ʌ m p θ ɪ ŋ]   [g oʊ w aʊ t]   [w i j i tʃ]
[n oʊ w oʊ l d ɚ] [ð i j i s t]   [s t r ɛ ŋ k θ] [t u w aʊ w ɝz]
[p æ n t θ ɚ]   [k ʌ m p f ɚ t]   [t u w i t]   [n oʊ w aɪ d i]

5. a. [ð i j i zi w eɪ j aʊ t]
   b. [ð ɪ s ː i m z oʊ k eɪ]
   c. [b ɛ t ɚs eɪ f n̩ s ɑ r i]

SPEECH RHYTHM AND SUPRASEGMENTAL ASPECTS

6. Primary accent:

[ˈn æ tʃ ɚ ḷ]   [s ə ˈs p ɛ k t]   [ˈd ɪ dʒ ə t ḷ]
[ɪn ˈf l eɪ ʃ n̩] [ˈs ʌ s p ɛ k t]   [r ɪ ˈw ɔ r d]
[ˈk oʊ b r ə]   [ɪn ˈs ʌ l t]   [ˈt i d i j ə s]
[ˈv ɪ d ɪ j oʊ] [ˈɪn s ə l t]   [k ə n ˈs ɛ n t ɪ ŋ]

7. Sentences—question/intent:

Statement	Question/Intent
a. <u>I'm</u> too busy to handle that now.	I'm even busier than usual.
b. I'm <u>too</u> busy to handle that now.	I might have time later.
c. I'm too busy to handle that <u>now</u>.	All I could do is look at it, not deal with it.
d. I'm too <u>busy</u> to handle that now.	I could handle a smaller, different task.
e. I'm too busy to handle <u>that</u> now.	Someone else might be able to do it.

8. Connected sentence transcription:

   a. [aɪ d oʊ n b i l i v ɪ t // aɪgɑ t n̩ eɪ]
   b. [oʊmaɪ / ɪ t s t aɪ m t ə g oʊ]
   c. [d ɪ dʒ ə h ɪr əbaʊtːæ t // aɪ d ɪ d n̩ t]
   d. [ð eɪ k eɪ m n̩ f ɝ s t n̩ s ɛ k n̩ d / r ɪ s p ɛ k t ə v l i]
   e. [p l i z b r ɪ ŋ m i ə p ɛ n / s ə m p eɪ p ɚ / n̩ ə d ɪ k ʃ ə n ɛ r i //]

9. Intonation:

   a. rising
   b. falling
   c. rising
   d. rising
   e. rising

CHAPTER 7

	/i/	/ɪ/	/e/	/æ/	/a/	/ɔ/	/o/	/u/
F1	300 Hz	400 Hz	600 Hz	700 Hz	750 Hz	600 Hz	600 Hz	400 Hz
F2	2300 Hz	2000 Hz	1900 Hz	1700 Hz	1100 Hz	900 Hz	900 Hz	1100 Hz
F3	3100 Hz	2800 Hz	2500 Hz	2400 Hz	2400 Hz	2400 Hz	2400 Hz	2250 Hz

Approximate formant frequencies for the first three formants (F1, F2, F3) for eight selected vowels, as estimated from Figure 7–9. Since these are estimated from a graphical representation, your answers might be as much as 100 Hz different from the ones shown here. Please re-examine any of your answers that are more than 200 Hz different from the ones shown in this table.

CHAPTER 8

1. Answers for exercise 1 in Chapter 8 will vary.
2. Regional dialects
   a. SE, ApE
   b. NEE, SE
   c. SE, ApE
   d. ME
   e. SE, ApE
3. African-American English
   a. meant   [m ɪ n]   e. burst   [bɜs]
   b. fine   [f ɑ̃]   f. shelf   [ʃ ɛf]
   c. other   [ʌdə]   g. birthday   [bɜfdeɪ]
   d. herself [hɜsɛf]   h. desk   [dɛks]
4. Hispanic English
   a. very   [bæri]   e. skirt   [ɛskɛrt]
       shovel   [tʃʌbl]   scurry   [ɛskɛri]
   b. breathe [brɪd]   f. call   [koʊl]
       Keith   [kɪt] or [kɪs]   law   [loʊ]
   c. choose   [ʃʊs]   g. ship   [tʃip]
       juice   [dʊs]   chip   [ʃip]
   d. which   [huiʃ]   h. thumb   [tɑm] or [sɑm]
       win   [huin]   sung   [sɑn]

CHAPTER 9

1. *Error transcription:*
   /k/ : t/k (I, M, F)   /g/ : d/g (I, M)   /tʃ/ : ʃ/tʃ (I, F)   /ʒ/ : -/ʒ (M)—d/ʒ (F)
   /θ/ : f/θ (I, F)—/θ/ (M)

2. *Phonological process usage:*

Target Word	Transcription	Final Consonant Deletion	Stopping	Velar Fronting	Gliding
cup	[t ʌ]	X		X	
rocket	[w ɑ t ɪ]	X		X	X
rake	[w eɪ]	X			X
gum	[d ʌ]	X		X	
wagon	[w æ d ə]	X		X	
pig	[p ɪ]	X			
sun	[t ʌ]	X	X		
bicycle	[b aɪ t ɪ t ə l]		X	X	
house	[h aʊ]	X			
shoe	[t u]	X	X		

INDEX

Italic page numbers refer to information in figures and tables.